World Health Organization (Ed.)

Benzodiazepines and Therapeutic Counselling

Report from a WHO Collaborative Study

With 48 Tables and 2 Illustrations

Springer-Verlag
Berlin Heidelberg New York
London Paris Tokyo

World Health Organization (WHO)
Avenue Appia
CH-1211 Geneva 27

Library of Congress Cataloging-in-Publication Data. Benzodiazepines and therapeutic counselling: Report from a WHO collaborative study / World Health Organization. p. cm. Bibliography: p.
ISBN-13: 978-3-642-73714-5 e-ISBN-13: 978-3-642-73712-1
DOI: 10.1007/ 978-3-642-73712-1
1. Benzodiazepines. 2. Mental illness–Chemotherapy–Evaluation. 3. Mental illness–Chemotherapy–Research. I. World Health Organization.
RC483.5.B48B45 1988 616.89'18–dc19

Softcover reprint of the hardcover 1st edition 1988

Typesetting
2125/3130-543210 – Printed on acid-free paper.

Contents

1 Introduction

1.1 Review of the Mental Health Programme of the World Health Organization (WHO)

Some 40 million people in the world are suffering at any one time from severe mental illness. Estimates of the number of people who are less seriously incapacitated by mental disorder vary, but none is lower than 200 million. In many countries, mental disorder is the main cause of disability in two out of every five disabled persons. Nearly one-fifth of all people seeking help in any general service suffer from some form of mental or psychosocial disorder. The size of the challenge is such that no progress could even be imagined without collaboration between the WHO member states and the productive involvement of the world's scientific community.

The World Health Organization cooperates with countries in formulating national mental health policies, in improving methods of the organization of care for the mentally ill and in developing techniques for the treatment and management of psychiatric illness (WHO 1982; Sartorius 1978). In these efforts, a variety of scientific disciplines and social service sectors have been involved (WHO 1981). The multisectoral and multidisciplinary approach of the programme is not only applied in dealing with the problems posed by mental disorders: equally so, this strategy is used in pursuing the other objectives of the programme, dealing with the promotion of mental health, prevention and control of drug- and alcohol-related problems, and psychosocial aspects of health and development in general.

In the field of psychopharmacology WHO's concern has focused on three main issues: first, on ways and means to ensure application of knowledge in the treatment of the mentally ill (WHO 1976); second, on research necessary to improve our knowledge about psychopharmacotherapy (Vartanian 1979 a); and, third, on the prevention of harmful public health consequences of psychotropic drug use and abuse (Harding and Chrusciel 1975).

The study which is described here belongs to the second of these areas of concern. As with its other research projects, the aims of the Organization are not only to obtain knowledge which can make the use of psychotropics safer and more effective but also to increase the research capacity of the centres participating in WHO-sponsored investigations (Vartanian 1979 b).

1.2 Related Efforts of the Organization

Until 1976 psychopharmacological research coordinated by WHO was restricted to the assessment of the effectiveness of drug treatment in the framework of other studies, for example, that on course and outcome of mental disorders in various populations (Sartorius et al. 1977; WHO 1979). Since then a more focused programme of psychopharmacological studies has been initiated (WHO 1980).

The origin of these studies was in the need to confirm or disprove the growing number of anecdotal reports about sizeable differences in the drug dosages necessary to achieve a good response by patients in different populations (Sartorius 1973). Reports from Africa and other tropical parts of the world refer to observations that doses of drugs such as chlorpromazine could be as low as half that used in the northern hemisphere and still achieve a full therapeutic effect. Similar findings or impressions have been reported for antidepressant drugs and tranquillizers.

It is hardly necessary to underline the tremendous scientific, practical and ethical impact that such a finding – if confirmed by well-controlled studies – could have on the theory and practice of psychopharmacotherapy and connected research. The evidence available to date allowed no definitive conclusions on this point, and consultation which WHO had with leading experts from a variety of countries did not result in any new data that could provide decisive help in this matter. All that was acquired were further accounts suggesting that people living in different climates and nutritional and sociocultural conditions need significantly different therapeutic dosages of commonly prescribed psychotropic drugs.

In view of this, WHO decided to undertake a multicentre collaborative research project for the assessment of the effects of psychotropic drugs in populations living in different sociocultural settings and differing in their way of life, ecological conditions and morbidity patterns. In selecting medicaments for the study the Organization was guided by two considerations: first, they should be medicaments which are widely used, and, second, they should be medicaments which have shown their effectiveness in the treatment of the most frequent mental disorders.

On the basis of these two criteria, three interrelated studies were launched: Dose Effects of Antidepressants (WHO 1986), Dose Effects of Neuroleptics, and Effects of Benzodiazepines and Therapeutic Counselling. Twelve collaborating centres participated in the studies. This report is concerned with the third of these studies.

In all three studies informed consent was requested of all subjects and was obtained according to local regulations. Conformity with accepted WHO guidelines was to be ensured, as was adherence to local ethical principles for medical research involving human subjects. These guidelines are based on the Helsinki Declaration I (of 1964), and II (of 1975), and have been drawn up by the WHO Secretariat Committee on Research Involving Human Subjects (SCRIHS).

1.3 Reasons for Undertaking a Study Using Benzodiazepines

Various minor psychiatric conditions, in which the dominant symptom is usually anxiety, are not only extremely common but are also often a source of disability and of a significant loss of working capacity. The treatment for these is usually some form of psychotherapy – ranging from intensive treatment based on psychodynamic theory, and lasting up to many years, to various forms of brief counselling, with or without adjunct treatment with psychotropic drugs.

Anxiolytic drugs are most frequently used, and the most popular among these are the benzodiazepines. They are used extensively all over the world, although there has been debate on their effectiveness as a treatment for anxiety states and on the dosage required. While the short-term efficacy of these drugs has been demonstrated, the benefits and hazards of longer term use are less well known although there is now a widespread recognition that a number of them have the propensity to produce dependence.

The study reported here is an international collaborative investigation using a comparative and prospective design to approach the question of the usefulness of benzodiazepine tranquillizers given in conjunction with and compared to therapeutic counselling for the treatment of minor psychiatric disorder.

The present study did not consider such essential uses of diazepam in developing countries as the management of tetanus, cerebral malaria, eclampsia and other emergencies of childbirth, and chloroquine and similar intoxications, and also as an adjunct to anaesthesia under adverse conditions (Ward 1985).

The study was undertaken in the context of primary care services since this is the context in which patients with anxiety syndromes are most often seen and given tranquillizers.

The centres in Bombay, Ibadan, London and Tokyo participated in the study throughout, from the point of designing the project to the agreement on the meaning of data and wording of the report.

1.4 Acknowledgement

This study is the product of a joint effort by many people. The original idea for the project came from Prof. N. Sartorius, and the first draft of the research protocol for the study was prepared by Prof. S. R. Hirsch in collaboration with Dr. F. E. Vartanian. It was further developed and finalized in collaboration with all the investigators and several temporary advisers. Numerous other individuals and institutions helped in the development of the protocol and in the conduct of the study. These included members of Expert Advisory Panel and Mental Health, heads of WHO Collaborating Centres in many countries and deans and directors of psychiatric medical institutions of centres mentioned below.

Dr. F.E. Vartanian, Senior Medical Officer, Division of Mental Health, WHO, Geneva, was the WHO officer responsible for the study and coordinated it from WHO headquarters in Geneva from 1979 to 1980. Mr. T. Ngo Khac, Technical Officer, assisted in the conduct of the study. Dr. N. Sartorius was responsible for the conduct of the study from 1980 until its completion.

The study was carried out by the teams in four centres; these are as follows:

Bombay: Prof. V.N. Bagadia (Head), Dr. P.V. Pradhan, Dr. I.R. Rajkumar, Ms. J.H. Gopalani

Ibadan: Prof. M. Olatawura (Head), Dr. A.O. Odejide, Ms. C.O. Ayinde, Ms. G.O. Awosika, Ms. R.O. Francis, Ms. B. Johnson, Ms. M.O. Tsekiri

London: Prof. S.R. Hirsch (Head), Ms. T.M. Mitchell, Ms. P. Turtin, Ms. P. Perry
In addition, the following General Practitioners participated in the study by allowing the investigators to see their patients: Drs. A. Bowden, S.J. Carne, A.E. Davidson, G.A. Dove, D.K. Fairweather, J.I. Koppel, J.E. Scriven and W.M. Styles

Tokyo: Prof. M. Kato (Head), Dr. Y. Nakagawa, Dr. Machizawa, Dr. T. Takahashi, Dr. Ogasawara, Dr. N. Takahashi, Dr. Kawamura, Dr. Shikiba, Ms. Kikuchi, Ms. Saito, Ms. Nakamura, Ms. Sasaki

Prof. Max Hamilton assisted in the analysis of the data and the preparation of the report. Prof. Olatawura prepared a review of the literature on which Chap. 2 was based. Data processing and statistical analysis were carried out at Vanderbilt University, Nashville, Tennessee, USA, under the supervision of Dr. W.H. Wilson. Ms. D.L. Appiah (WHO headquarters) has conscientiously, carefully and patiently prepared the many drafts of this manuscript.

The project was initiated with the full cooperation of the collaborating centres and with significant support from F. Hoffmann-La Roche and Co., who also provided and packaged free of charge diazepam (Valium Roche) and placebo tablets.

2 Literature Review

2.1 Literature on Cross-Cultural Comparisons of Effectiveness of Psychotropic Drugs

As early as the late 1950s and early 1960s it was recognized that wide discrepancies occurred in the dosage of phenothiazines prescribed in British, French and Swiss hospitals. It was thought that these dissimilarities could be a function of differences in diagnosis, criteria for clinical change, treatment setting, staff attitudes, environmental pressures, drug manufacture or diet (Denber 1960). As information about clinical experiences with psychotropic drugs from different parts of the world became known, interest in the effects of psychotropic drugs in different populations grew tremendously, particularly in the past 15 years or so. A review of the literature shows that many of the factors earlier thought to influence the differences in drug dosages are still largely relevant.

Okuma (1981) noted that of the many variables which determine the effects and side effects of psychotropic drugs, the *host factor* is one of the most important. A lower sensitivity of schizophrenics compared with normals to the sedative effect of chlorpromazine was demonstrated quantitatively by a higher percent time of waking EEG in the schizophrenics following medication. In a transcultural context, the mean therapeutic dose of chlorpromazine for the manic state was found to be much lower in Japanese than in Western populations, in a controlled study comparing the antimanic efficacy of carbamazepine and chlorpromazine. Itil (1975) demonstrated similar differences between psychiatric patients and normal volunteers given different psychotropic drugs. Denber et al. (1962) compared the effectiveness of butyrylperazine in psychotic patients in Manhattan State Hospital (United States) and in Erlangen (Federal Republic of Germany) and discovered that the Manhattan State Hospital patients required five times the dosage of butyrylperazine to achieve the same therapeutic effect as those in Erlangen. It was striking that the patients in the United States receiving much heavier doses developed 30% fewer extrapyramidal effects.

After their finding that Hispanic depressed patients required about half the dosage required by white patients in New York for comparable therapeutic results, and that the Hispanic patients complained of more side effects, Marcos and Cancro (1982) urged that apart from pharmacokinetic factors, psychological, sociocultural and biological characteristics of patients should be considered when interpreting similar results.

The transcultural significance of the host factor with respect to differences in therapeutic plasma level was demonstrated by the study of Yamashita and Asano (1979). These workers showed that although Asian depressed patients tended to respond to lower doses of antidepressants when compared with American depressed patients (1.4–2.7 mg/kg compared with 3.5 mg/kg body weight) this was not related in a simple way to steady-state plasma levels of the tricyclics. In general terms, despite the low dosage corresponding to low plasma levels, Asian patients showed the same therapeutic response as American patients on much higher plasma levels. Takahashi et al. (1979) found the same trend with respect to patients receiving lithium for affective disorders in Japan and the United States. Ghoneim et al. (1981) demonstrated that clear ethnic differences exist in the mental effects and kinetics of diazepam between Caucasians and Orientals. Total body clearance was higher in Caucasians than Orientals to a significant degree while serum concentrations of desmethyldiazepam were higher in Orientals.

The influence of the host factor in explaining some of the differences in drug requirement and drug response in different cultures is further highlighted by the known sites of drug metabolism in the mammalian body, particularly the liver. The case of slow versus rapid metabolism of various drugs has been explained on the basis of genetic differences (Cosmides 1970). In general terms, genetic enzyme defects may cause specific drug toxicity. Forrest et al. (1975) directed our attention towards agents such as pesticides and food additives which induce drug-metabolizing hepatic enzymes. Chlorinated pesticides are very generously used in farming and animal husbandry in North America. North Americans are known to drink substantial amounts of milk and consume more animal fats, which store more of these compounds, than do people in the rest of the world.

Other factors thought to contribute to the prescription of higher drug doses include the induction of hepatic microsomal drug-metabolizing enzymes by other drugs. Drugs known to increase microsomal protein and induce additional drug-metabolizing enzymes include barbiturates, diphenylhydantoin, diphenylhydramine and various steroid hormones. Certain drugs may speed their own metabolism when given chronically to the extent that increasing doses must be given to achieve the same desired therapeutic effects. In a series in the United States, 30% of chronic schizophrenics also suffered from associated alcoholism, with gastric complaints or sleep disturbance. These patients may receive antacids or barbiturate sedatives in addition to antipsychotic medication. Barbiturates cause increased urinary excretion of chlorpromazine, due presumably to additionally induced drug-metabolizing enzymes, while antacids, due to absorption phenomena, interfere with chlorpromazine absorption (Forrest et al. 1970).

In summary, while Booij (1975) has drawn our attention to the biochemical individuality of the human organism, the host factor in mediating differences in drug response (therapeutic or side effects) would appear to be a function of the differences in such variables as body weight, diet, climate, personality factors (including alcohol use and smoking), genetic differences and previous exposure to drugs that include barbiturates, alcohol and nicotine (Raskin and Crook 1975; Kortilla et al. 1976; Olatawura 1977).

Quite apart from the host factor, another variable that has been shown to account for differences in the response pattern of patients from different cultures is the psychopathological symptom profiles of the study subjects. In their comparative study of the effectiveness of butaperazine on schizophrenics in Istanbul (Turkey) and Missouri (United States), Itil and Reisberg (1977) found that the Turkish patients had a better response and at a lower dosage than did the schizophrenics in the United States. Moreover, the Turkish patients who received lower doses of antipsychotic medication showed more side effects than did those in the United States. The authors were quick to point out that although the 'typical' symptoms of schizophrenia of the Turkish and the American patients were similar, the Turkish patients had more florid symptoms such as agitation, hallucinations and delusions compared with the patients in the United States. Also, the American patients were more chronic in that they had had longer courses of medication and higher dosage histories with other psychotropic drugs compared to the acutely presenting Turkish patients. In their cross-cultural study of antidepressant agents carried out in the United States and Bogota (Columbia), Escobar and Tuason (1980) also indicated that patients from developing countries showed a better response to antidepressants compared with American patients. They noted that Columbian patients showed greater psychopathology, a factor also thought to account for the greater placebo response of the Columbian patients.

Another important factor thought to contribute to the differences in psychotropic drug responses in different cultures is that of the measuring instruments employed by investigators. In their study of psychiatric patients in Italy and the United States by means of common measuring instruments, namely the Inpatient Multidimensional Psychiatric Scale (IMPS) and the Johns Hopkins Check List, Crane (1966) showed that measuring instruments not sensitive enough to tap culturally loaded symptoms can give different results even when used by the same researchers in two different cultures. For example, the Italian raters compared with their American counterparts showed the greatest difference in rating the syndrome of somatization. The Italian raters tended to give higher ratings to symptoms of somatization compared to American raters, even though the coefficient of correlation between the two raters was high. The study also demonstrated that a difference in the assessment of a patient's psychopathology seems to be more related to the type of patient examined and/or the rater's personal bias than to a basic difference in the scientific background of the psychiatrists trained in two different countries. It also showed that results obtained by European psychiatrists using doses of phenothiazines which investigators in the United States would consider homeopathic may be due to a selection of patients with relatively mild mental disorders.

Simeon (1975), after reviewing the methodological problems inherent in evaluating therapeutic responses in different cultures, suggested that valid ratings can be obtained by using a behavioural rating scale only if the psychiatrist is thoroughly familiar with the patient's culture and can empathize with him. Even then, he advised that transcultural psychopharmacology should avoid diagnostic categories heavily dependent on social and cultural values where the biological integrity of the organism is presumably preserved, such as in neuroses and personality disorders. This methodological problem is less significant with entities on which it is easier to agree, such as schizophrenia and affective and organic psychoses.

In summary, even though Ban et al. (1974) found that there was no difference in the effectiveness of clomacran between a North American population and a Mexico City patient population (despite differences in cultural background and initial psychopathology), there is impressive evidence that there are differences in the effects of psychotropic drugs in different populations. Some of the factors shown to account for these include the host factor, the types of patients studied, and the measuring instruments employed to collect data on study subjects as well as to measure the therapeutic and side effects of the drugs. A recent comprehensive review by Lin et al. (1986) subdivides host factors into cultural, genetic (which show themselves through variations in metabolism) and environmental. They also indicate what further work should be done on these factors.

The Benzodiazepines. Epidemiological studies have shown that there is a high prevalence of mental diseases in developing as well as in developed countries. A WHO Joint Study has confirmed that the percentage of mental disease varies between 10.5% and 17% among adults of the areas studied; for children the levels range between 11% and 29%. The majority of adults presented with neuroses, while among children behaviour disorders and mental retardation were most common. It has been established that minor affective disorders are common among patients consulting general practitioners (Goldberg and Blackwell 1970; Goldberg et al. 1976). These disorders present mainly with symptoms of anxiety or depressed mood, and often with a mixture of the two (Goldberg and Huxley 1980; Shepherd et al. 1981). General practitioners commonly prescribe psychotropic drugs, mostly benzodiazepines, for these minor affective disorders.

In discussing the role of benzodiazepines in the psychosocial aspects of mental health care in developing countries, Busnello (1979) indicated that "in the case of neurotic patients and those presenting chronic complaints basically of an emotional nature, the benzodiazepines figure as a powerful aid in health problems of populations in developing countries on account of their ease of management, safety, efficacy and efficiency". The benzodiazepines form part of a list of 15 essential drugs, drawn up by the WHO, thought desirable to be 'mastered' and available to primary health care workers in the context of extending mental health services to the community. The benzodiazepines deserve special consideration as psychotropic agents because of the magnitude of neurotic disorders in all communities, both developed and developing countries, of the world and because of the widespread use of benzodiazepines by both professional and auxiliary health workers to treat minor affective disorders, amongst others.

There are two pertinent questions that deserve greater examination. First, how safe are benzodiazepines and, second, how really effective are benzodiazepines in view of the fact that many of the minor emotional conditions for which benzodiazepines are freely prescribed may either be self-limiting or improve rapidly with non-professional intervention such as chatting with a friend or one's priest. With regard to the first question, Ladewig (1983, 1984), Winokur et al. (1980), and Petursson and Lader (1981) have shown that benzodiazepines are widely abused. Benzodiazepines exhibit partial cross-tolerance vis-à-vis all the substances belonging to the alcohol barbiturate type of drug dependence. Several other possible dangers of benzodiazepines reported include increased proneness to road-traffic accidents (Betts et al. 1972; Seppala et al. 1976), hostility and paradoxical reactions (Hall and Joffe 1972; Salzman et al. 1974; British Medical Journal 1975), interaction with alocohol (Hayes et al. 1977) and contribution to self-poisoning (Hawton and Blackstock 1976). Williams et al. (1982) showed that 20% of patients in the United Kingdom who were prescribed benzodiazepines continue to take them after 6 months. Regarding self-poisoning, one of the remarkable properties of the benzodiazepines is their safety when taken in acute overdosage (Prescott 1983).

As for the effectiveness of the benzodiazepines, the evidence is mixed. Some writers have reported that they may be valuable in general practice for minor affective disorders (Wheatley 1975; Priest 1980). However, there are studies suggesting that a placebo may be just as effective as anxiolytic medication for low levels of anxiety (Rickels and Downing 1970; Dasberg and van Praag 1974). In a carefully controlled study of the effects of non-prescribing of anxiolytics for patients usually given benzodiazepines by general practitioners, Catalan et al. (1984a, b) sought to answer four questions. The answer to the question, "Does withholding anxiolytic drugs prolong psychological distress that might have been relieved by anxiolytic medication?" was clearly negative. The answer to the question,"Does withholding anxiolytic medication increase the consumption by patients of other substances?" was also negative. There were no reported increases in the use of alcohol, tobacco or non-prescribed drugs. With regard to the question, "Does withholding anxiolytic medication fail to fulfil the patients' expectations?" no significant difference was found between the group given anxiolytic medication and the group not given it. The final question about whether withholding anxiolytic medication made unreasonable demands on general practitioners' time showed a negative answer. While these findings support the results of previous studies (Goldberg and Blackwell 1970; Kedward 1969) which had established that a substantial proportion of this type of patients recovers rapidly with brief counselling, Catalan et al. (1984a, b) further demonstrated that patients who are poor responders by the end of 1 month tend to have more severe initial and persistent anxiety/depressive symptoms. They are also distinguished by the use of alcohol and tobacco.

The issues raised above, namely the widespread use of benzodiazepines for minor emotional problems in general practice, the undoubted dangers of their unsupervised use, the fact that in many instances patients traditionally given benzodiazepines did not suffer when they were withheld, as well as the fact that they are being advocated for use in primary health care makes the WHO-sponsored comparative study of benzodiazepines and brief psychotherapy in different cultures timely and its results of particular importance.

2.2 Literature on Cross-Cultural Comparisons of Psychotherapy

Psychotherapy has been variously defined but the following definition will serve our present purpose. Psychotherapy is a therapeutic processs of psychological interaction between the therapist and the patient. The therapist's main mode of helping the patient is by creating a setting in which the patient can talk about his or her problems and the therapist's response, as well as the patient's response to the therapist, are important elements in the treatment.

When the therapist comes from the same culture as the patient the problem of communication is reduced to a considerable extent. However, there are other equally important components of psychotherapy which influence cross-cultural comparisons. One is perception by the therapist of dysfunction in the patient who consults him with the aim of seeking relief from his problems. It can sometimes be difficult to distinguish what is cultural from what is psychopathological. The patient may show exaggerated cultural traits that cross the barrier between cultural adaptation and psychopathological dysfunction. Also, the external reality, stresses and defences of a patient may be such as to interfere with his ability to benefit from insight-oriented psychotherapy. In this regard, the material socioeconomic stresses of patients are, in many places, particularly in the poor countries of the world, so pressing that a precipitate examination of conflicts and characteristic coping style of the patient might be considered an inappropriate step. Such patients usually need concrete help to alleviate their material distress before they can benefit from insight-oriented psychotherapy (Olatawura 1976).

One other important factor of cross-cultural relevance is motivation. As has been pointed out by Bluestone and Vela (1982), patients whose complaints are externalized (e.g. "If my son would behave well I would have no problems") or whose problems are somatized to multiple organs (as is often the case with neurotic patients from developing countries), with little awareness of something psychologically wrong, will have limited motivation for insight-oriented psychotherapy. Another factor of importance which can affect motivation is a patient's expectation when he visits the doctor. Wood and Sherrets (1982) studied the importance of obtaining medication as a reason for contacting an out-patient psychiatric service from the perspectives of white and black patients. Blacks were found to attach greater importance to getting medication than whites. Commenting on folk medicine versus biomedicine among the Chinese, Kleinman (1981) noted that "like many non-western peoples, patients in China and Taiwan regard injections as the most potent and therefore most desirable form of western medicine". As a result they frequently demand injections for sicknesses that they regard as serious, regardless of the type of medicine prescribed.

Transference and countertransference phenomena correctly identified and properly handled facilitate the resolution of the patient's problems. Traditional child-rearing practices foster the development of excessive dependence and inhibition of aggression in children in traditional societies (Benfari 1969). This trait carried into adulthood may result in the patient seeing the therapist as someone who can gratify him. The patient in psychotherapy may thus become passive and expect the therapist to solve his problem for him (Bluestone and Vela 1982).

Finally, Schlesinger (1981) has drawn our attention to the influence of culture on the goals of psychotherapy. In his opinion, the goal of therapy for the Asian patient is to enable the individual to fit into the family unit and into society at large in an appropriate fashion. Normative standards of behaviour are derived culturally. The points raised above lend tremendous support to the conclusion of Krause and Howard (1983) that, as far as design and analysis issues in cross-cultural evaluation of psychotherapies are concerned, psychotherapies and cultures cannot be made experimentally independent because important input processes and outcome variables essentially involve participants' meanings and feelings, which are not naturally invariant across cultures.

2.3 Literature on Methodological Issues Involved in the Conduct of Comparative Studies

The issue of the validity of data collected in the course of cross-cultural studies has rightly received due attention in the literature (WHO 1973; Simeon 1975; Ulett and Ulett 1975; Davies et al. 1975; Joyce 1975, 1980; WHO 1979). Although the problem is quite complex, the following points, which are relevant to a discussion of validity in any study, acquire added significance in cross-cultural studies:

1. Reliability and validity of assessment instruments
2. Obtaining a homogenous sample of subjects
3. Expectations of the study population (for example, regarding the form of medication in drug trials and expectation of quick results)
4. Getting reliable measures of change so that recorded changes are perceived as having the same meaning from centre to centre
5. Inferences drawn from the data collected

Murphy (1969) has stressed the influence of culture on symptomatology, psychopathology and the extent of inhibition, vigilance and intrapsychic complexity in individuals. Thus all the elements of reliability in any study, namely the interviewers, the schedules, the raters and the respondents, are subject to complex cultural influences in multicentric trials of drugs for psychiatric conditions (Hamilton 1975).

Rickels (1968) gives an account of the effects on the outcome of therapy of such factors as the setting of the consultation and the expectations of patient and therapist. Joyce (1980) has stressed the need to take account of the influence of factors which he referred to as 'non-specific' on the specific effects of drugs on individuals participating in drug studies. These include the constitution (physical and psychological) of the individual, his acquired characteristics (immunity, expectation, experience) and his environment. The latter includes people (doctor, staff, family, friends and fellow patients), the disease, nutrition, climate and social drugs such as alcohol and nicotine. Because of the compounding effects of 'non-specific' factors on specific drug effects, Joyce (1980) believes that within-country studies hold a better promise of producing more valid results than between-country studies. Despite the undeniable reality of complex methodological problems in the conduct of cross-cultural studies, it is widely accepted that such studies can make valuable contributions to the issues of diagnosis, course and outcome of psychiatric disorders. Taking collaborative studies as an example, Sartorius (1983) has articulated the step-by-step approach designed to improve the validity of cross-cultural research data.

2.4 Literature About Administrative/Procedural Aspects of Multicentric Trials

The difficulties that characterize administrative and procedural aspects of multicentric trials can be identified in all aspects of any such trial. They affect the recruitment of the study subjects, the measuring instruments and the treatment modality (drug or psychotherapy) being evaluated. Murphy (1975) has drawn our attention to a common but often overlooked source of bias, namely, the process by which the patient reaches the clinician or researcher. With some patients, years can elapse between the onset of symptoms and the first contact with a psychiatric service, while other patients seek and obtain attention within a few weeks. Another related origin of differences between cultures is the recruitment source of study subjects. In this regard, Wheatley (1975) has pointed out the difference between domiciliary and institutional trials. Patients in general practice are unsupervised and the reliability of drug taking may be influenced by this factor. In a cross-cultural context, institutional trials pose special problems in developing countries. These include shortage of infrastructural facilities, particularly beds, which restricts admission to hospital to the most seriously ill, a factor that in itself leads to a high turn-over of patients. Other factors that affect hospital admission and attrition rates, include long distances of patients from hospital and economic constraints, especially, as is often the case in developing countries, when patients have to pay for their treatment.

Other factors of importance have been amplified by Wheatley (1975) and they include the influence of cultural norms on diagnosis, differing professional customs and conditions of medical practice, differing therapeutic customs, dietetic habits, social codes and customs, public reaction to mental illness, and the living and working conditions of the different populations. As an example of the influence of living and working conditions on the outcome of trials, the provision or lack of good welfare services may be crucial. It has been argued that there is less incentive to return to work if high unemployment benefits are available and this may affect response to treatment in psychoneurotic illness.

The problems posed by the influence of language on measuring instruments were highlighted earlier; so were the problems due to the attitude of different cultural groups towards injections as opposed to tablets and capsules influencing compliance and ultimately the results of cross-cultural drug trials. It is known that psychotherapy as developed and practised in Western cultures has its special problems in the developing countries. Joyce (1975) has identified two main interrelated factors affecting the methodology and outcome of multicentric drug trials. They are language and ideas. These can interact in various ways. Firstly, concepts may be the same while the language is different; secondly, the language may be the same while concepts are different between centres; and, thirdly both concepts and language may be different between centres. The WHO has demonstrated that many of these administrative and procedural aspects of multicentric collaborative research posed by concepts and language are not insurmountable (WHO 1973).

3 Aims of the Study

The aims of the study were:

1. To determine the short- and medium-term efficacy of minor tranquillizers for patients presenting to physicians with a wide range of minor physical and psychological symptoms including mild depression, tension, anxiety and worry, and to compare them with no treatment (placebo) and with brief counselling of a sort which might be given by non-psychiatrists in medical practice.
2. To determine whether the effects of these compounds are only short lived (2 weeks) or persist over a 6- to 12-week period, as compared to placebo.
3. To see if there is a wide variation among different populations in the effects and unwanted effects at different dosages.
4. To determine the effect of the clinician's decision to discontinue treatment or not after 6 weeks, as determined by the 12-week outcome of patients treated with these compounds.
5. To consider the relationship between life-events and response to treatment.

4 Description of Materials and Methods

4.1 Design of the Study

In each centre the treatments formed a two-way factorial design: drugs at two levels (absent and present) and psychotherapy at two levels (counselling and no counselling; Fig. 1). Once the patients were included they were randomly assigned to one of the four groups thus defined. The four centres added a third dimension to the design. Clinical assessments were made at the start of the trial (week 0), at week 2 and at week 6. Every effort was made to complete all the assessments. For example, if the patients did not attend for evaluation, an attempt was made to visit them in their home. The repeated observations thus formed a fourth dimension in the design. Although counselling was a factor which crossed all the other three, individual counsellors worked only in their own centre and thus were 'nested' within centres, i.e. the 'effects of counsellors' cannot be separated here from those of centres.

The trial ended formally after the 6th week, but it was then left open to the physicians to continue treatment for another 6 weeks. At the end of this period, further assessments were made.

4.2 Description of Centres at Which the Study Took Place

The study involved four centres, in developing and developed countries: Bombay (India), Ibadan (Nigeria), London (United Kingdom) and Tokyo (Japan).

An important part of any research, one which influences the results obtained and their interpretation, is the selection of subjects for study. Multicentre studies present problems because of the likelihood of differences in population samples from one centre to another. This may lead to differences in results and thus present problems in interpreting the results. In this study the four populations studied have been selected precisely because they are different – from racial, cultural and socioeconomic points of view. However it would be possible to interpret the effect of cultural differences on the outcome of the study, even if the subjects were in all other respects similar, only if the samples of the patients selected at each centre were similar in terms of diagnosis, prognosis, attitude for treatment etc. For example, if studying patients with grade I carcinoma of the breast it could be said that the patients were similar in respect to diagnosis and prognosis and other variables could be considered as having an independent effect on the outcome of breast cancer. This is not the case in our study because it is not possible to determine with the same certainty that the clinical condition

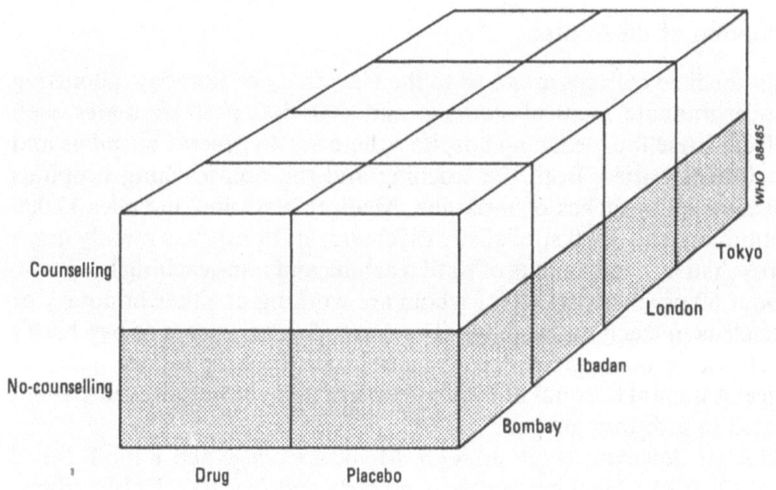

Fig. 1. Design of Trial

studied, or the reason for patients' coming for help, is the same from one centre to the next. The present study has been designed to investigate the value of brief, simple counselling, of benzodiazepine medication, and of a combination of the two in patients presenting themselves to a primary care, direct-access medical facility where out-patients come with a variety of minor medical disorders. The null hypothesis that these treatments have no effect was tested separately in four centres with different ethnocultural populations. A combined analysis was also undertaken to look for treatment effects independent of the treatment centre and population differences.

4.2.1 Description of Research Centre and Study Area of Bombay

4.2.1.1. Description of Catchment Area

Bombay is a cosmopolitan, metropolitan island in western India with a total area of 433.71 km^2 and an ever-increasing population of 8 243 000. The average population density is 18 333/km^2, but in the southern part of the city the density is 47 810/km^2 – one of the highest in the world.

Textile, chemical, pharmaceutical, engineering, oil, metal and fertilizer industries predominate, and it is here that 55% of the population are employed. Shortage of housing is a major problem: 80% of the city's inhabitants live in one-room tenements. As the city is geographically linear, transportation is difficult. People living in the north and working in the south travel 2–4 h daily. The literacy level is 68%, as compared to 36% in the whole of India.

4.2.1.2 Description of the Centre

There are four medical colleges attached to the University of Bombay, admitting some 600 undergraduate medical students and 400–500 post-graduates each year. Apart from these four teaching hospitals there are 40 general hospitals and 130 municipal dispensaries. Both the teaching and the non-teaching hospitals have specialists in all branches of medicine. Medical personnel includes 12000 general practitioners and 3000 specialists. Psychiatry in Bombay is mainly organized in the psychiatric departments of both teaching and non-teaching hospitals. There are about 60 psychiatrists, 20 of whom are working as either honorary or full-time specialists in teaching hospitals. There are 15 departments of psychiatry with about 210 beds; out-patient departments in all the hospitals provide for walk-in service. A mental hospital of 1000 in-patients and with a daily out-patient clinic is situated in a distant suburb.

The Psychiatric department of Seth G.S. Medical College and King Edward VII Memorial (K.E.M.) Hospital provides 60 beds and has 1000–1100 admissions per year. Daily out-patient clinics cater to about 7000 new and 38000 repeat consultations per year. The types of treatment given in the Department are psychopharmacotherapy, electroconvulsive therapy, brief psychotherapy of a problem-oriented and supportive type, behaviour therapy, group educational therapy, family case work, educative counselling, child guidance therapy and occupational therapy.

Referrals from other branches of medicine, consultation-liaison psychiatry, is part of the routine activity of the Department. Nearly one-third of patients are referred by other medical departments. Teaching of undergraduate medical students, training of post-graduate students in psychiatry, teaching of nurses, physiotherapists, occupational therapists and psychiatric social workers also belong to the routine activities of the Department.

The research conducted here is largely clinical and consists of psychosocial and phenomenological study of major and minor psychiatric conditions including psychosomatic disorders such as diabetes mellitus and mucous colitis. Treatment research is a regular feature and consists of evaluation of psychopharmacotherapy, electroconvulsive therapy, psychotherapy, behaviour therapy etc. in various psychiatric conditions. Schizophrenias, depressions, alcoholism and neuroses are the four major conditions which receive priority in research. Newer areas of research include the detection and management of psychiatric problems in out-patients attending medical, dermatological, gynaecological and obstetric, and otorhinolaryngological services, as well as a study of dying and death-related problems.

4.2.1.3 Recruitment of Patients

All patients attending the psychiatric out-patient service of our Department and diagnosed as suffering from minor psychoneurotic problems were seen by a senior resident, and each was given the Need-for-Treatment Scale. Only those patients needing minor anxiolytics and/or counselling and not needing hospitalization or antidepressants were interviewed. Those living far away from the Department, those who could not come for regular evaluations as required, those already on psychotropic drugs, or those with alcohol or drug problems were excluded. The GHQ was administered to the remaining patients by the researcher, and those scoring 12 or more were included in the study.

4.2.1.4 Counsellor's Training and Experience

After graduation in economics, the counsellor at the Bombay centre had post-graduate training for 2 years at Nirmal Niketon, the College of Social Work at the University of Bombay. After obtaining the Master's Degree, she joined the Psychiatric Department of K.E.M. Hospital in 1970 where she has since been working as a psychiatric social worker. She has also supervised the students specializing in psychiatric social work from the Tata Institute of Social Sciences.

Apart from diagnostic work in collecting social data, she has actively participated in case conferences. From the very beginning she has been involved in therapeutic work (e.g. social case work), individual psychotherapy, group psychotherapy, therapeutic counselling with all age groups, family therapy, therapy with children with behavioural problems, group psychotherapy with relatives of children with behavioural problem, and relatives of patients given electroconvulsive therapy.

She has also actively participated in a number of research projects as co-author: drugs versus psychotherapy in depressive patients; a prospective and retrospective study of 300 children with behavioural problems; psychopathology in patients suffering from obessional-compulsive neurosis, writer's cramp and hyperhidroses; social therapy in schizophrenic patients; a study of *Cannabis indica*; psychopathology in alcoholic patients on aversion therapy; a study of the effect on children of schizophrenic patients; psychopathology in patients suffering from anxiety; and a comparative study of treatments for anxiety (behaviour therapy, drugs and psychotherapy). Recently, she has been involved in a psycho-social study of patients exposed to methylisocyanide in Bhopal, conducted by Dr. P. V. Pradhan, Honorary Associate Professor of Psychiatry, K.E.M. Hospital. Six papers have been published by her in the *National Journal of Indian Psychiatry*.

4.2.2 Description of Research Centre and Study Area of Ibadan

4.2.2.1 Description of Catchment Area

The city of Ibadan has a population of about 1.5 million people, mostly Yorubas, and is the administrative centre of one of the 19 states which make up the Federal Republic of Nigeria. Ibadan has both urban and "sub-urban" characteristics. The urban sector is characterized by the presence of government offices, business premises, industrial establishments, private property and educated white-collar workers. The sub-urban sector is occupied by the predominantly poorer and illiterate populations whose main source of income includes subsistence farming and low-paid jobs in offices and factories. The unemployment rate is about 10% of the potential labour force. The marriage pattern is polygynous. Traditional households or family compounds are very common in the suburban sector, while the urban sector is characterized by single-room lodgings for single clerks and apartments of up to three bedrooms for the more affluent married office workers.

4.2.2.2 Description of the Centre

The Ibadan centre is located in the Department of Psychiatry of the teaching hospital of the University of Ibadan, the oldest Nigerian university. The Department has considerable experience of participating in WHO multicentric collaborative studies, starting in the late 1960s with the International Pilot Study of Schizophrenia. The research staff thus have considerable experience with research instruments such as the PSE and the GHQ, which have featured in many WHO collaborative studies.

4.2.2.3 Recruitment of Patients

The patients admitted to this study were selected from the General Out-Patient Department of the teaching hospital. Using the Need-for-Treatment scale, the general-duty doctor who assigned patients to the specialist clinics each morning passed patients judged by him to have minor neurotic disorders to the research staff, who were also in attendance during the assignment stage. The patients were referred as they met the inclusion criteria, i.e. on a consecutive basis. Patients so identified were brought to the research psychiatrist in the Department, only a short distance from the General Out-Patient Department. The final decision to admit a patient to the study was made by the psychiatrist using the agreed inclusion criteria.

The two research psychiatrists in this project had had extensive experience in the use of both the full and short versions of the PSE. The research assistants were nurses whose basic training and work experience included both general and psychiatric nursing. In addition, two of the research assistants participated in the training exercises which took place in Copenhagen as well as in the reliability exercises which took place in London during the course of the study. The GHQ assessments and the counselling and its rating were done by the research assistants, while the research psychiatrists conducted the PSE.

4.2.2.4 Counsellors' Training and Experience

The two counsellors from Ibadan had their basic training and work experience in both general and psychiatric nursing. They were thus quite familiar with the processes of forming a therapeutic relationship with patients. These two counsellors had also participated in research interviews for an average of 10 years before starting the present study.

4.2.3 Description of Research Centre and Study Area of London

4.2.3.1 Description of Catchment Area

The study was carried out through four general practices, dealing with a mixed population ranging from skilled working class to upper-middle class. Patients here are usually seen by appointment but emergency cases are also seen during office hours.

4.2.3.2 Description of the Centre

The academic Department of Psychiatry has five full-time academic staff, including a professor, two readers and two lecturers. There are also five consultants and six trainees. There are nearly a dozen research workers and external students on research grants.

The Department has 40 beds, sees out-patients and does consultations for medical and surgical wards. There is also a day hospital. Patients are referred from their general practitioners, accident and emergency departments or other out-patient departments.

4.2.3.3 Recruitment of Patients

Patients were either referred by their general practitioner, in whose opinion they were suitable, or through identification from their scores on the GHQ which they completed while sitting in the waiting room.

The patients completed the GHQ themselves and the counsellors carried out the PSE and other assessments. Thus, the counselling treatments were not assessed blindly.

4.2.3.4 Counsellors' Training and Experience

The counsellors were a social worker with a diploma in social work and a social sciences graduate with much research experience. The former had had over 5 years experience in a department of psychiatry, and the latter had had much experience in counselling posts.

4.2.4 Description of Research Centre and Study Area of Tokyo

All the patients attending psychiatric out-patient services of Kohnodai National Hospital, a general hospital, and two private psychiatric hospitals were screened by psychiatrists with the Need-for-Treatment Scale. Those thought to be suffering from minor psychiatric complaints or having a possible emotional component were asked if they would participate in the study if it was thought that they might respond to counselling or benzodiazepine. If so, they were given the GHQ and randomized to counselling or non-counselling. Those assigned to counselling were referred to a clinical psychologist after the psychiatrist had administered the GHQ, PSE and other instruments. The psychologists had had a formal training of two years and 5 years or more counselling experience. In the event, some patients assigned to counselling dropped out before the evaluation, presumably because of the resistance that Japanese have to this kind of treatment.

4.3 Description of Samples and Manner of Selection

Patients were drawn from medical clinics or general practices in each country. They were new cases who had initially reported with physical or minor emotional complaints. They were selected in three steps on the basis of agreed criteria and then randomly allocated to one of the treatments.

4.3.1 Description of Samples

There were 296 male patients (48%) and 321 female patients (52%) in the total sample of 617. The greatest discrepancies were in Bombay with 24% female patients and in London with 71% (see Table 1). The mean age of patients was 31.3 years, ranging from the youngest at 13 (in Bombay) to the oldest at 77 (in London) (see Table 2). Overall, 15% of patients came from minority groups, although there was no information on 13% (see Table 3). The overwhelming majority were of urban origin, 69% coming from the centre of towns and 28% from the periphery (see Table 4). The majority (56%) lived in nuclear families, with little variation between the different centres regarding this (see Table 5). Their economic status (on a scale of: 1, lowest; 3, average; 5, highest) was close to the average for each respective country, but there were great differences between the countries from a social, economic and cultural perspective (see Table 6). Educational backgrounds varied considerably: 58% in Ibadan were illiterate, while 5–12 years of schooling was reported by 59% in Bombay, 63% in London and 39% in Tokyo (see Table 7). The majority of patients were employed, but there was considerable variation, with Ibadan showing the highest proportion (65%) of self-employed persons. In Tokyo 49% were classified occupationally as 'other', signifying housewives, pensioners, students, etc. (see Table 8). Physical illnesses were reported in previous years by 14%; 15% had had previous mental illness, thus indicating that 85% came for treatment during their first attack (see Table 9). Within the centres, the demographic characteristics of the different treatment groups were very much the same (differences were not statistically significant). This applied even in London where, of the 16 female patients who received counselling, six were given diazepam, and of the 32 who did not receive counselling, 18 were given the active drug. It is clear that centres differ considerably from each other, and it could be expected that this may lead to very different results.

The diagnosis of 84% of patients was anxiety state but again there was considerable variation between centres. All but one of the 209 cases in Bombay were diagnosed as anxiety state (International Classification of Diseases, 300.0), but in Ibadan the corresponding rate was 92%, with another 6% diagnosed as neurotic depression (300.4). The corresponding figures for London were 66% and 20%, with a further 9% diagnosed as neurasthenia. The figures for Tokyo were 44% and 13%, respectively (see Table 10). In every centre a physician agreed that the patient was suitable for entry into the trial. Diagnoses were not necessarily made by a psychiatrist or physician but may have been made by a research worker who was trained as a social worker and worked in psychiatry. Psychiatric assess-

Table 1. Sex

	Bombay		Ibadan		London		Tokyo		All centres	
	n	%	*n*	%	*n*	%	*n*	%	*n*	%
Men	159	76.1	68	34.3	48	29.1	21	46.7	296	48.0
Women	50	23.9	130	65.7	117	70.9	24	53.3	321	52.0
Total	209	100	198	100	165	100	45	100	617	100

Table 2. Age of subjects

	Bombay	Ibadan	London	Tokyo	All centres
Mean	24.98	33.14	35.53	37.18	31.31
Lowest	13	17	15	17	13
Highest	45	50	77	62	77
n	209	198	165	45	617

Table 3. Majority and minority groups

	Bombay		Ibadan		London		Tokyo		All centres	
	n	%	*n*	%	*n*	%	*n*	%	*n*	%
Majority group	89	42.6	170	85.9	142	86.1	41	91.1	442	71.6
Minority group	48	23.0	28	14.1	18	10.9	0	0.0	94	15.2
Missing information	72	34.4	0		5	3.0	4	8.9	81	13.1
Total	209		198		165		45		617	

Table 4. Type of residence

	Bombay		Ibadan		London		Tokyo		All centres	
	n	%	*n*	%	*n*	%	*n*	%	*n*	%
Rural	10	4.8	1	0.5	0	0.0	2	4.4	13	2.1
Urban peripheral	82	39.2	57	28.8	10	6.1	24	53.3	173	28.0
Urban central	115	55.0	138	69.7	153	92.7	19	42.2	425	68.9
Other	1	0.5	0	0.0	1	0.6	0	0.0	2	0.3
Missing information	1	0.5	2	1.0	1	0.6	0	0.0	4	0.6
Total	209		198		165		45		617	

Table 5. Type of household

	Bombay		Ibadan		London		Tokyo		All centres	
	n	%	*n*	%	*n*	%	*n*	%	*n*	%
Nuclear	102	48.8	103	52.0	114	69.1	25	55.6	344	55.8
Extended vertically	22	10.5	63	31.8	2	1.2	12	26.7	99	16.0
Extended horizontally	25	12.0	24	12.1	1	0.6	6	13.3	56	9.1
Extended both ways	1	0.5	3	1.5	1	0.6	2	4.4	7	1.1
Missing information	59	28.2	5	2.5	47	28.5	0	0.0	111	18.0
Total	209		198		165		45		617	

Table 6. Socioeconomic status

	Bombay	Ibadan	London	Tokyo
Mean	2.33	2.34	3.12	3.07
n	209	197	165	45
Missing information	0	1	0	0

Table 7. Education

	Bombay		Ibadan		London		Tokyo		All centres	
	n	%	*n*	%	*n*	%	*n*	%	*n*	%
Illiterate	20	9.6	114	57.6	0	0.0	0	0.0	134	21.7
Literate, no school	4	1.9	1	0.5	1	0.6	0	0.0	6	1.0
5 years of school	21	10.0	36	18.2	1	0.6	1	2.2	59	9.6
5–12 years of school	123	58.9	38	19.2	104	63.0	17	37.8	282	45.7
12 years, no University	30	14.4	4	2.0	31	18.8	19	42.2	84	13.6
University graduate	8	3.8	2	1.0	21	12.7	6	13.3	37	6.0
Post-graduate	2	1.0	0	0.0	4	2.4	0	0.0	6	1.0
Vocational school	0	0.0	0	0.0	1	0.6	1	2.2	2	0.3
Other	0	0.0	3	1.5	1	0.6	0	0.0	4	0.6
Missing information	1	0.5	0		1	0.6	1	2.2	3	0.5
Total	209		198		165		45		617	

ments were not carried out in terms of a psychiatric medical interview. Thus, the diagnostic differences between centres, as reported in this study, reflect the diagnostic and labelling practices of those making research-diagnostic decisions at each centre as much as it does the relative proportion of patients with a particular pattern of symptoms at each centre.

Table 8. Working status

	Bombay		Ibadan		London		Tokyo		All centres	
	n	%	*n*	%	*n*	%	*n*	%	*n*	%
Self-employed	23	11.0	129	65.2	6	3.6	3	6.7	161	26.1
Employed	97	46.4	40	20.2	114	69.1	15	33.3	266	43.1
Unemployed	25	12.0	10	5.1	12	7.3	3	6.7	50	8.1
Sick leave, employed	0	0.0	0	0.0	1	0.6	1	2.2	2	0.3
Sick leave, unemployed	2	1.0	0	0.0	1	0.6	1	2.2	4	0.6
Other	6	2.9	1	0.5	31	18.8	22	48.9	60	9.7
Not applicable	56	26.8	18	9.1	0	0.0	0	0.0	74	12.0
Total	209		198		165		45		617	

Table 9. Past physical and mental illness

	Bombay		Ibadan		London		Tokyo		All centres	
	n	%	*n*	%	*n*	%	*n*	%	*n*	%
Past physical illness	14	6.7	15	7.6	40	24.2	16	35.6	85	13.8
Missing information	0	0.0	2	1.0	4	2.62	1	2.2	7	1.1
Past mental illness										
None	189	90.4	195	98.5	113	68.5	28	62.2	525	85.1
Out-patient	11	5.3	0		40	24.2	12	26.7	63	10.2
In-patient	1	0.5	0		6	3.6	2	4.4	9	1.5
In- and out-patient	0	0.0	0		1	0.6	1	2.2	2	0.3
Other treatment	0	0.0	0		0	0.0	1	2.2	1	0.2
No treatment, evidence of illness	1	0.5	0		1	0.6	0	0.0	2	0.3
Missing information	7	3.3	3	1.5	4	2.4	1	2.2	15	2.4
Total	209		198		165		45		617	

4.3.2 Manner of Selection of Patients for the Study

4.3.2.1 Criteria for Inclusion

At the first interview, selection for admission into the trial took place in three stages:

1. Patients had to have the type and severity of illness appropriate to the investigation, i.e. they were identified as having emotional components in their complaints, for which the doctor thought that benzodiazepines, counselling or both could be a suitable treatment. This could include mild depression. The criteria for this would differ from centre to centre.
2. Patients had to conform to the requirements for attendance, i.e. they had to live sufficiently near to be able to come for treatment, did not suffer from physical

Table 10. Diagnosis[a]

		Bombay		Ibadan		London		Tokyo		All centres	
		n	%	*n*	%	*n*	%	*n*	%	*n*	%
Anxiety states	300.0	208	99.5	183	92.4	109	66.1	20	44.4	520	84.3
Hysteria	300.1			1	0.5	1	0.6	1	2.2	3	0.5
Neurotic depression	300.4	1	0.5	12	6.1	33	20.0	6	13.3	52	8.4
Neurasthenia	300.5			1	0.5	15	9.1	4	8.9	20	3.2
Hysterical personality disorder	301.5					1	0.6			1	0.2
Phobic state	300.2							2	4.4	2	0.3
Obsessive-compulsive disorder	300.3							3	6.7	3	0.5
Depersonalisation syndrome	300.6							1	2.2	1	0.2
Hypochondriasis	300.7			1	0.5			6	13.3	7	1.1
Unspecified	300.9							2	4.4	2	0.3
Missing information		0		0		6	3.6			6	1.0
Total		209		198		159		45		617	

[a] International Classification of Diseases (9th edn.)

illness which would prevent attendance, and were willing to return at 2–12 weeks for follow-up.
3. Patients had to have a minimum score of 12 on the GHQ, administered by a member of staff.

4.3.2.2 Criteria for Exclusion

Patients excluded from the study were the following:
1. Patients requiring antidepressant or neuroleptic medication, or those thought to be suffering from a severe depressive or psychotic illness.
2. Patients thought to have any kind of major physical illness, such as malaria, amoebiasis, influenza, etc., or any other physical conditions affecting their general health, i.e. those thought to be too physically ill to be suitable for the study.
3. Patients who had an established history of alcohol or drug dependence.
4. Patients living beyond a radius of easy accessibility for the research worker, as determined in each centre.
5. Patients who were unlikely or unwilling to come for 2-week, 6-week and 3-month follow-ups.

4.4 Description of Instruments Used for Assessment and Training of Research Workers

Information was collected in the course of five interviews and up to six counselling sessions. Data were recorded in the patient documentation file for each patient. Administrative forms included the General Practitioner's Rating – Need for Treatment Scale, the Demographic Description (day 0), and the Personal Treatment Record (each time a prescription was made).

There were four meetings of investigators and a training seminar before the study began. These gave the centres and research workers ample opportunity to rehearse the use of scales. A further meeting held while the study was in progress confirmed that there was good agreement between raters in using the GHQ, PSE und RSSE. Two systematic differences between centres in the use of the Audit of Counselling scale emerged. The first was in the inclusion of 'general conversation' as part of the counselling process in some centres but not in others. The second was in the varying use of the intervention categories, 'history taking' and 'exploration' in some centres and 'exploration' and 'ventilation' in others. In future studies a more explicit operational definition of these categories should be provided.

The following forms were completed for the assessment of change: GHQ on days 0, 14, 42 and 84; RSSE on days 0, 14 and 42; PSE on days 0 and 12; and the Brief Life Events Questionnaire (BLEQ) on days 42 and 84.

Counselling was recorded on the Audit of Counselling forms at the end of each counselling session and when the patient's counselling treatment had been completed. In summary, the study schedule was as follows:

Study Schedule

Form	Screen	Week			
		0	2	6	12
Need-for-Treatment Scale	×	×			
General Health Questionnaire	×		×	×	×
Demographic Description	×	×			
Present State Examination		×		×	
Audit of Counselling[a]		—	—	—	—
Final Audit of Counselling[b]		—	—	—	—
Rating Scale for Side Effects		×	×	×	
Personal Treatment Record[c]		—	—	—	—
Brief Life Events Questionnaire				×	×

[a] Repeated after each counselling session
[b] Completed when counselling finished
[c] Completed each time a prescription was made

4.4.1 General Health Questionnaire (GHQ)

The GHQ has been used to detect minor psychiatric morbidity among patients attending general practices in the United Kingdom (Goldberg 1972; Goldberg and Hiller 1979) and the United States. It normally is given as a self-administered questionnaire consisting of 60 items on a four-point scale scored 0, 0, 1, 1 (maximum score, 60). This method is that usually referred to in the literature. This was used for screening purposes (the Screening Score), a score of 12 or determining eligibility for this trial; in Japan, however, the cut-off level was 11 points. For analysis of the outcome of treatment, the Likert method was used, assigning values of 0, 1, 2, 3 to positions on the four point scale (maximum score, 180); a 0 score on a particular item means that there is no change from usual, and 3 means that the patient feels much worse than usual. Thus, patients with a chronic complaint may score 0 (not different from usual) when they have been suffering the symptoms for a long time. For the purpose of this study, which focuses on the efficacy of pharmacotherapy and psychotherapy for recently emergent minor disturbances, this limitation of the GHQ does not have great importance.

The English version of the GHQ was translated into three local languages in India (Hindi, Gujarathi, Marathi), one language in Nigeria (Yoruba) and into Japanese. Back translations were carried out. The local versions were then modified according to the comments received on the back-translated versions.

Goldberg and Hiller (1979) conducted a factor analysis on the resulting data, using a varimax rotation on the first four principal axes (factors). Two of these factors are of particular relevance to this investigation: 'anxiety and insomnia' (consisting of items 14, 18, 39, 44, 45, 47 and 55) and 'social dysfunction' (items 21, 22, 28, 30, 35, 36 and 42; see Appendix B).

In addition to the GHQ, information was gathered on the patient's physical state, as assessed by the research worker. These data contain information on height, body weight, pulse rate and blood pressure. It should be noted that if the patients were illiterate, the research worker questioned them and filled in the questionnaire accordingly.

4.4.2 Present State Examination (PSE)

The PSE schedule is a guide to the structuring of a clinical interview, with the object of obtaining a valid and reliable description of the present mental state of adult patients suffering from one of the functional psychoses or neuroses. The schedule was developed in the early 1960s, and the first eight editions were tested extensively (Wing et al. 1967; Kendell et al. 1968; Cooper 1970). The ninth revision of this research instrument (that used here) has been shown to have adequate reliability both at the level of observation and when combining symptoms to syndromes (Wing et al. 1974). It is available in some 20 different languages and has been used extensively in many studies.

The PSE consists of 140 symptoms and can be administered by a trained psychiatrist in 30–90 min, depending on the number of symptoms the patient exhibits. PSE ratings give global assessments covering the absence or presence, in moderate or severe symptomatology, over the past month, but when the scores are summed, there is a strong correlation with the GHQ (above 0.8) due to a large non-specific general factor common to all psychiatric disturbance (Newson-Smith and Hirsch 1979). In the present study, however, the time referred to has been limited to the past 2 weeks. The resulting score sheets were provided in the patient documentation file to be used in conjunction with the PSE interview schedule.

Further work on the reliability of the PSE (Wing et al. 1977) has shown that for individual symptoms the kappa coefficient ranges from 0.34 for free-floating anxiety to 0.84 for depressed mood. Total scores obtained at the same interview give an inter-rater reliability of 0.73 (Pearson's correlation coefficient).

4.4.3 Rating Scale for Side Effects (RSSE)

Treatment-emergent symptoms (side effects occurring during the course of treatment) are recorded on the RSSE, originally developed by Asberg et al. (1970) and adapted for this study. For improving reliability, some of the definitions of symptoms and their gradation were suitably modified. In addition, two items – 'interference with sexual functioning' and 'other symptoms considered during interview to be important' – were introduced. The scale consists of seven items and two ratings were required for each symptom: spontaneously reported manifestation and systematically checked symptom. By using a rating before starting the treatment it was possible to separate somatic manifestations from real side effects presumed to be due to medication.

4.4.4 General Practitioner's Rating – Need for Treatment Scale

A special instrument for selecting patients was prepared. This contains the ratings for the two stages during the screening procedure: the section on the General Practioner's Rating – Need for Treatment Scale ensured that patients had the type and severity of illness appropriate to the investigation; the section on 'further information', included only patients who met the requirement for attendance. Personal data of the patients, i.e. sex, age and marital status, are also recorded for those patients who have fulfilled the criteria for inclusion.

The instrument was administered to those patients for whom the general practitioner had time to fill out the scales and at out-patient clinics.

4.4.5 Demographic Description

The Demographic Description instrument was designed to collect, as far as possible, data describing the economic, social and cultural characteristics of the study populations to illustrate the background of the patients who were selected and assessed. It also provided information about past physical and mental illnesses of the patients (see Tables 1–10).

4.4.6 Brief Life Events Questionnaire (BLEQ)

Previous studies have suggested that the rate of occurrence of life events is correlated with the precipitation of psychiatric syndromes (Brown et al. 1973 a, b; Day 1981). The BLEQ was designed to collect information on events that had happened to the patient in the past 3 months, or up to 2 years if the problems were still present. The purpose of this instrument was to determine whether there are any relationships in these populations between the presence of stressful life events and the persistence of symptomatology of minor psychiatric disorder. It consists of 21 items, grouped under seven problem areas, and also contains the ratings on 'independence of events'. The BLEQ does not conform to the requirements of a more intensive study of the role of life events as carried out by Brown and Harris (1978), although it was derived from their methodology.

The seven subsections of the BLEQ are: illness/injury, schooling, work, finances, relationships, children/family and other changes/losses. The form was completed at weeks 6 and 12 on the basis of an interview by the research assistant.

4.4.7 Personal Treatment Record

The Personal Treatment Record recorded all treatments given to the patients during the 12 weeks of the clinical trial, with an indication of the dosage, the frequency and reason for clinical decision. Entries were made each time a prescription was made.

4.4.8 Audit of Counselling

The Audit of Counselling instrument was developed to provide a quantitative method of characterizing the nature of counselling as given at each centre, in terms of what the patient was being counselled about, how the counsellor conducted the sessions technically, what the counsellor felt was most important, and progress which the counsellor felt had been made.

The schedule is composed of two parts. Part A consists of the Quantitative Description of Interview, which was to be filled in immediately after each counselling session. This part is divided into four sections:

1. Basic data necessary for the identification of the patient.
2. A rating scale to determine what the subjects dealt with in the session. The investigator estimated the percentage of time he/she spent on any of these particular problems.
3. The technique used by the counsellor and its importance within the interview. The investigator used his/her best estimate of the importance and percentage of time which he/she spent using a particular technique.
4. The counsellor's assessment of the quality of client–counsellor interaction to identify how the patient reacted within each counselling session.

Part B consists of the Final Audit of Counselling and Retrospective Assessment of Change, filled in when the patient's counselling treatment had been completed. This part was also included if counselling consisted of two or more sessions, either when counselling had finished or when the patient had dropped out. This part is divided into three sections:

1. Identification of the patient.
2. The importance and progress achieved for each problem area discussed during the interview. The counsellor rated his/her judgement of the overall importance of any problem area leading to the patient's distress. Progress was divided into the areas of objective change, consisting of the counsellor's rating of actual changes in the patient's circumstances (e.g. improved housing conditions, reduced number of arguments with spouse) and subjective change, consisting of changes in the way in which the patient felt about the problem(s) (e.g. housing or sexual problems may or may not have been improved, but the patient nevertheless felt better or worse about it).
3. The counsellor's overall evaluation of the patient's improvement and the contribution of counselling to it.

4.5 Treatments

4.5.1 Choice of Drugs and Dosage

Diazepam is thought to be the most widely used minor tranquillizer in most countries throughout the world and was chosen for this reason. This drug is now listed in the pharmacopoeia and can be produced by any manufacturer. It was essential that a placebo be employed in the study, as the spontaneous remission rate for minor psychiatric disorders, although unknown for developing countries, is certainly considerable in northern Europe. A placebo was also given to provide a baseline for comparison with pharmacologically active substances.

Diazepam was prescribed in the form of 2-mg tablets three times a day for a minimum of 2 weeks. The dosage could then be increased, if required,to a maximum of 12 mg daily. Placebo tablets were prescribed in similar quantities. The patients were further allocated to groups receiving counselling or not. Thus the four treatment groups provided a completely balanced research design.

In the event, there was no significant difference in the dosage of drug given to the two counselling groups, at any time or in any centre. After the 2 weeks of fixed dosage differences appeared, and from the 4th week on, the dosage in Bombay (over 8 mg daily) was significantly higher ($p < 0.001$) than in the other three centres (6–7 mg/day). This continued to be true for the periods up to weeks 6 and 12. Although the mean dose given to the non-counselling group was always greater than to the counselling group, none of the differences reached a statistically significant level (see Table 45).

It must be noted that at week 12, these data were only recorded for 137 of the 212 patients receiving the drug, with the majority (55%) of these in Ibadan.

4.5.2 Counselling

The counsellors were advised to give counselling as often as they thought necessary. It was recommended that for the first two sessions this might be up to 1.5 h and for the remaining ones 15–30 min. At the end of each session the counsellor recorded a quantitative description of the interview, and after the final session the final audit and retrospective assessment of counselling was recorded.

4.5.2.1 Description of the Counselling Process Employed at the Bombay Centre

Counselling at the Bombay centre was given according to the recommendations of the study protocol. The first two sessions were, as far as possible, more restricted to data collection and exploration which helped to identify the patients' major difficulties and primary sources of dissatisfaction. The problems identified were then discussed in the remaining four sessions. Goals of treatment were selected according to information available, on a priority basis. Although the first goal of treatment was to bring symptomatic relief, the intermediate and immediate goals were taken care of in the counselling process.

Specific goals for counselling were unique to each client. Consequently, the counselling process was shaped by considerations of these goals. Techniques and design procedures were then adopted to facilitate their accomplishment.

The counselling process was conducted in a structured and permissive relationship, with the aim of helping patients to gain an understanding of themselves and to improve their decision-making skill to enable them to take positive action and make behavioural changes. Two types of counselling were offered in most of the cases, related to the kinds of patients referred: (a) crisis intervention and (b) facilitative counselling. The latter counselling was used most effectively in clarifying the patients' thinking; helping them with self-understanding and acceptance; devising a plan of action by working together; and, finally, acting in a responsible manner by enhancing their ego-capacity. Reassurance was found to be a more effective technique in patients with prolonged illness and psychosomatic-type symptoms. With patients who had already developed vague fears and misconceptions about their illness in the initial stage, it was difficult for the counsellor to convince the patients that their illness was psychogenic. It was especially important to take care of this factor as it had further aggravated their already existing anxiety symptoms.

The first two sessions, as mentioned above, were restricted to history taking. The patients were encouraged to talk or ventilate their feelings. Using techniques served the following purposes:

1. It gave the counsellor sufficient scope to understand the psychopathology of the patient and to formulate the goals.
2. At the same time it helped the patients to abreact their feelings by showing sympathy, warmth, permissiveness and acceptance, which helped to establish the positive rapport and mutual trust between counsellor and patient. This relationship between counsellor and client was effectively used in subsequent sessions in achieving the desired change in the patient's behaviour or in helping the patient to accept the situation.

The concerns in counselling included, for example, choosing academic options, planning a career, improving interpersonal relationships with family members and with fellow workers, helping to find out potential capacities, interests and aptitudes, as well as helping them to recognize the 'why' of their behaviour, its self-defeating nature, but yet their doing nothing to change it. There was no pre-established time schedule for achieving the goal, but the process was directed or designed to facilitate goal attainment; simultaneously, goal formation was also influenced by the clients' expectations.

Most of the time the discussions focused on the present and future. As far as possible the patients were discouraged from talking about their past, as the counselling was oriented toward immediate goals, and revival of the past would not have helped, except in some cases where to talk about the past was relevant to the present difficulties.

Resistant and defensive patients were handled tactfully, and after the development of a rapport they were encouraged to talk in general terms; this ultimately helped the counsellor to understand those aspects of the situation which he had neglected or had not realized by denying the appropriate consideration. The counsellor's task here was to keep the patients on the track and to give attention to neglected aspects.

After total identification as to how the counsellor could best help the patients to change, and what the patients expected of him or her, the appropriate technique was decided. Care was taken that problems were discussed and worked out together. Advice giving was used cautiously and economically in subsequent sessions when sufficient rapport had been established. Although history taking and exploration were restricted to the first two or three sessions, reassurance and interpretation was combined, i.e. in sex-anxiety cases.

The patients were given 'patient listening' to ventilate their feelings as well as to understand their problems and attitudes, thus helping to direct the progression of the interview. Interpretation was most frequently used when it was helpful to the patients in gaining insight into the cause and effect of their symptoms, in view of their life conflicts. Reassurance was used when patients with a long duration of problems expressed vague fears and concepts about their sickness. This technique was found more useful and effective in sex-anxiety cases.

Challenge was used only when the patient showed hysterical overlay, and when there was secondary gain to maintain the symptoms. In some of the cases, when the patient used defences such as denial or intellectualizing the situation, challenge was used cautiously. Some of the patient's resistance was overcome by perseverance coupled with tactful questioning and exploration, without insisting that the illness was psychogenic. This happened with those patients where pathology was not clear-cut or obvious.

The improvement response was slow in patients with (a) severe, continuing life stress and conflicts, (b) hysterical overlay, (c) long duration of symptoms, or (d) psychosomatic symptoms. There was gradual and slow improvement, with occasional intercurrent relapses, in patients with long duration of pathology and continuing severe psychopathology in life situations.

4.5.2.2 Description of the Counselling Process Employed at the Ibadan Centre

One of the aims of counselling in this study was to identify problem areas that might be responsible for patients' neurotic symptoms. The first session, as practised at the Ibadan centre, was spent mainly on obtaining a good history. The patients, seated in a quiet room, were given ample time to discuss their symptoms as they perceived them. In particular, patients were asked to describe their understanding of the origins of their symptoms. It is usually of prognostic importance to differentiate those patients who ascribe their symptoms to witchcraft from those whose symptoms are not compounded by such fears. In addition, specific probes were directed at areas such as money, housing, work and marital relations. In this regard, particular attention was focused on the problems associated with polygyny and the extended family system. In the case of married female patients, they were asked whether they were the only wive or one of several. If the latter was the case, they were asked how they got on with other wives, how much financial support was forthcoming from the husband, whether they were living with their husband under the same roof, and, if not, how frequently they saw their husband. Married male patients were asked, amongst other things, whether they had problems with their wives, and, if so, what the nature of the problems was.

Problems associated with the extended family system were also systematically probed. Patients were asked whether any relatives were living with them, and what this meant in terms of over-crowding, family budget and having to cope with other demands stemming from the extended family members. Patients were also asked whether they were supporting elderly parents or the education of cousins. These are some of the usual demands of the extended family system on members who are of working age. At the end of the first session, part A of the Audit of Counselling, i.e. Quantitative Description of the Interview, was rated according to the problem areas identified. The percentage of time spent on each problem area and the rapport established by the counsellor were noted.

With this baseline, counselling took place at 2-week intervals. The specific approach depended on the problems of the patients. In general, counselling took the form of exploration of patients' complaints, getting patients to ventilate their feelings, encouraging or reinforcing a desirable style of coping, giving advice when desirable, and increasing the insight of patients by interpretation. At the end of each session a record of what had transpired during the session and the length of time spent on each aspect of the patient's identified problems was noted in part A of the Audit of Counselling (Quantitative Description of the Interview).

Completion of part B, i.e. the Final Audit of Counselling and Retroactive Assessment of Change, took place on the 6th visit, or on the 3rd or 4th in the case of patients who dropped out of the study at these earlier stages. At this final stage the counsellor assessed the importance and the progress achieved for each problem area. In particular, the counsellor was interested in determining how successful the patients were in relating their initial symptoms to the identified problems. Finally, the counsellor estimated the contribution of counselling to the improvement observed.

4.5.2.3 Description of the Counselling Process Employed at the London Centre

At the London centre patients were told at the point of referral to the project researcher that they would be given the opportunity of six short counselling sessions. The first two interviews were the longest, being up to 1.5 h in total. The remaining sessions were very brief – about 15 min. The aim of the sessions was to help patients gain a better understanding of their problems and of why they had got themselves into difficulties. The counsellor could help them to pinpoint certain areas of difficulty when they themselves perhaps felt overwhelmed by distress and were unable at that time to see how they could change things. The counsellor could serve the purpose of aiding the clients to clarify their problems and could assist them in trying to change, for example, regarding recurrent patterns of behaviour that brought dissatisfaction to them.

A hypothetical example of this: A man came to the general practitioner with tension headaches. It was revealed he had just been abandoned by his girl-friend who was married and several years older than he. During counselling it was demonstrated to the patient that he had created a pattern of functioning that was bound to be destructive to him. He had had several affairs with married women, usually being the hurt partner when the relationship broke up. He began to understand through counselling that he was terrified of commitment and marriage (having witnessed several bad marriages when he was a child) and became entangled in relationships with women which unconsciously he sensed would never materialize, thus not having to become emotionally committed.

In this study patients were usually referred to the counsellor for somatic symptoms, e.g. sleeplessness, unexplained back or chest pain, general fatigue. This was not surprising as the patients were seeking help from a primary health care setting where the expectation was for them to have a health problem rather than an emotional disorder.

The patients would already have had opportunities to talk about their symptoms by the time they came for counselling because a PSE would have been administered. Counselling therefore usually took the form of helping the patients gain a better understanding about their behaviour and to view their problems from an angle different from hitherto. Counselling might be of a purely supportive nature, for example, to bolster the patient's spirits and confidence. Sometimes it was found useful to set goal targets; this meant that by a certain date the patients would have completed agreed tasks.

The counsellors expressed the opinion that the short period of time allotted to counselling in this study did not allow for work of real depth to be undertaken, but that useful work could be done in the minimal time given if the patients were motivated for change and willing to accept help. Often the patients were reluctant to see the counsellor because they feared being branded as neurotic.

4.5.2.4 Description of the Counselling Process Employed at the Tokyo Centre

The counselling method most frequently applied at the Tokyo centre was an indirect, passive one, most similar to the Rogers' method or Morita therapy. Very few therapists here use the psychoanalytical approach.

Counsellors in Japan felt that they needed more time than allotted. This was due mainly to two reasons. First, the Japanese, as a homogeneous race, share a common religious, moral, linguistic and behavioural background. Therefore, human inter-relationships are group-dominated, and each person is aware of his fellow humans' thinking and behaviour because they reflect his own. Thus, a counsellor would hesitate to delve deeply into a patient's secrets unless the patient voluntarily spoke out on the problem. Knowing exactly how the other person would feel can be a drawback.

Second, neurotic patients in Japan are less expressive than their Western counterparts, in particular on the question of sexual and marital problems. On the other hand, they are very sensitive when treated experimentally, a fact which may be linked to their lack of confidence towards the doctors and also towards the drugs used. However, they seldom express this lack of confidence directly with the doctor, but simply stop attending the clinic.

These attitudes may be almost the same in the counselling process, and although the patient rarely argues with the doctor, they may move to another clinic. Additionally, almost all private practitioners deliver drugs directly to the patient rather than prescribing them through a pharmacist, as was the procedure in this study.

A number of patients in Japan refused to enter the trial, and among those who did enter a proportion refused to accept counselling as a method of treatment. An additional complication was that patients who were dissatisfied with their progress normally moved to another doctor.

The first session took 1–2 h, during which topics discussed were general (history-taking). The counsellors were passive listeners, and the patient's speaking out was emphasized. Sensitive discussions were avoided, especially on questions which the patients would have been likely to avoid (e.g. sexual or marital secrets). The reason that such sensitive areas as the patient's secrets and problems were avoided at the first session was to form a better doctor–patient atmosphere. This was particularly true if the patient seemed to be intentionally avoiding these issues.

The second session took place 2 weeks after the first. The contents of counselling were approximately the same as in the first session. From the viewpoint of the counselling process, patients could be divided after the second session into three groups. In the first group, patients' speaking out had seemed to be a catharsis, and patients were on the way to recovery. The second group of patients rejected the counsellor and wanted to terminate the project. The third group of patients (which was very small) were defensive and yet showed an interest in what the counsellor was doing; they were not open-minded. For this group of patients a more intensive or psychoanalytical approach was deemed appropriate.

5 Results

The first step in the analysis of the data is to examine the effects of randomization to determine whether any systematic biases have been introduced. It is customary to do so by submitting various data such as means or distributions to a test of statistical significance. If, for example, the means of the randomized groups differ, the test may show that the differences are 'significant'. This means that if the groups had been randomly sampled from a population, then the means would have differed by as much or more a given percentage of the times. In fact, we know that they *were* randomly sampled, so it is legitimate to ask what the statistical test is doing. It is giving information on the differences of, for example, the means in terms of standard units, which makes it easier to judge how large are those differences. It will then be necessary to decide whether the difference can be ignored, or should be eliminated by using the variable under consideration as a covariant in an analysis of covariance. If the distributions differ considerably, it may be necessary to use appropriate weights for the frequencies when carrying out later statistical tests.

In the event, no biases were found in the Bombay and Ibadan centres, but in Tokyo 32 out of 45 patients were allotted to no counselling (Table 11). However, the counselling groups were proportionately divided among the drug and placebo groups. The overall χ^2 analysis indicated that there was a uniform distribution of patients across all centres.

The findings in London were that male patients were more frequently allotted to no-counselling (32 cases) then to counselling (16 cases), while the reverse was true for female patients, with 51 to no-counselling and 66 to counselling ($p=0.04$). Patients who had been allotted to placebo and no-counselling had

Table 11. Number of patients assigned to treatments in each centre

Centre	Treatment group										
	DWC		DNC		PWC		PNC		Total		χ^2
	n	%	*n*	%	*n*	%	*n*	%	*n*	%	
Bombay	49	23.4	56	26.8	47	22.5	57	27.3	209	33.9	0.718
Ibadan	52	26.3	48	24.2	47	23.7	51	25.8	198	32.1	0.172
London	41	24.8	45	27.3	41	24.8	38	23.0	165	26.7	0.298
Tokyo	6	13.3	15	33.3	7	15.6	17	37.8	45	7.3	4.294
	148		164		142		163		617		1.176

The low value of χ^2 shows that the randomization of patients to the four treatments is close to proportional, assessing even distribution. *DWC*, diazepam with counselling; *DNC*, diazepam with non-counselling; *PWC*, placebo with counselling; *PNC*, placebo with non-counselling

Table 12. Numbers of patients in each treatment group at the end of each assessment period and percentage of baseline admission

		Treatment group									
		DWC		DNC		PWC		PNC		Total	
		n	%	*n*	%	*n*	%	*n*	%	*n*	%
London											
Week	0	41	100.0	45	100.0	41	100.0	38	100.0	165	100.0
	2	38	92.7	43	95.6	41	100.0	36	94.7	158	95.8
	6	37	90.2	43	95.6	41	100.0	36	94.7	157	95.1
	12	24	58.5	34	75.6	29	70.0	20	52.6	107	64.8
Bombay											
Week	0	49	100.0	56	100.0	47	100.0	57	100.0	209	100.0
	2	42	85.7	47	83.9	42	89.4	46	80.7	177	84.7
	6	35	71.4	44	78.6	33	70.2	40	70.2	152	72.7
	12	33	67.3	30	53.6	29	61.7	29	50.9	121	57.9
Ibadan											
Week	0	52	100.0	48	100.0	47	100.0	51	100.0	198	100.0
	2	48	92.3	46	95.8	42	89.4	43	84.3	179	90.4
	6	40	76.9	43	89.6	38	80.9	37	72.5	158	79.8
	12	39	75.0	40	83.3	32	68.1	32	62.7	143	72.2
Tokyo											
Week	0	6	100.0	15	100.0	7	100.0	17	100.0	45	100.0
	2	6	100.0	13	86.7	7	100.0	10	58.8	36	80.0
	6	6	100.0	13	86.7	7	100.0	6	35.3	32	71.1
	12	1	16.7	11	73.3	1	14.3	4	23.5	17	37.8
All centres											
Week	0	148	100.0	164	100.0	142	100.0	163	100.0	617	100.0
	2	134	90.5	149	90.9	132	93.0	135	82.8	550	89.1
	6	112	75.7	143	87.2	119	83.8	119	73.0	493	79.9
	12	97	65.5	115	70.1	91	64.1	85	52.1	388	62.9

Table 13. Distribution by treatments of patients who remained or dropped out by week 6

	Treatment group				
	DWC	DNC	PWC	PNC	Total
Remaining	112	143	119	119	493
Dropped out	36	21	23	44	124
Total	148	164	142	163	617

$\chi^2 = 13.25$; $p \leqq 0.05$

stayed in their present residence for an average of 10.7 years, which is longer than for the other treatment groups (range 5.0–8.6 years). This difference was significant below the 0.02 level. As the standard deviations increase correspondingly with increasing means of this variable, it is likely that the frequency distribution of this variable is log-normal and that a suitable transformation would diminish the differences between the means of the four groups. The difference in the mean socioeconomic status of the four treatment groups was of only decimal magnitude and although statistically significant ($p < 0.0002$) had no clinical importance.

Bias may also be introduced by differences in the rate of drop-outs. Examination of the data (Tables 12 and 13) shows that up to 6 weeks the drop-out rates were all less than 30%. For all the centres together, the majority of drop-outs came from the group placebo with no counselling while the fewest were from that with diazepam with no counselling. It is worthy of note that in Japan it is customary for patients who are dissatisfied with their treatment not to hesitate to leave their physician for another; this probably accounts for the high drop-out rate in Tokyo. It is likely that the relatively poor results of 'treatment' in the placebo and no counselling group accounts for its many drop-outs; if so, this would bias the results by diminishing the differences between active treatment versus controls.

As the physician had the option of stopping the study treatment at the end of 6 weeks, it is difficult to evaluate the further losses by the end of 12 weeks, especially as the patients remaining in the trial by that time accounted for a mere 52%–70% of the original set of patients.

Correlations between scores on the BLEQ and those on the GHQ (used as a criterion of change; see Table 40) were found to be consistently low, ranging from −0.04 to +0.21, indicating that the relationship was weak, and that there would be no point in using BLEQ scores as a covariant in the analysis. (A more detailed analysis of the data on life events will be published separately.)

The correlation of GHQ scores, for all the centres, between weeks 0 and 6 was 0.35, and that between weeks 0 and 12 was 0.34. These low correlations provide indirect evidence that changes in the amount of improvement differed considerably from patient to patient. However, the correlation between weeks 6 and 12 was 0.61, indicating that much of the variability took place in the first period.

At the screening, scores on the GHQ did not differ significantly between the treatment groups within the Bombay, Ibadan or London centres (Tables 14–16). In Tokyo (Table 17), although the drug-treated group (mean, 29.5; SD, 13.77) did not differ significantly from the placebo group (mean, 24.9; SD, 11.17), the counselling group (mean 34.6; SD, 13.14) was higher than the no counselling group (mean, 23,9; SD, 11.03; $p < 0.01$; maximum possible scores, 180). With this one exception it would appear that randomization produced four groups of effectively similar patients, as measured by their scores.

5.1 Assessment of the Value of Instruments Used

As described in Sects. 4.3.1 and 4.3.2, the PSE and GHQ have been used for many years and been found to be of adequate reliability and validity. Joint training and

Table 14a. Screening and total scores, General Health Questionnaire: Bombay

Period			Treatment group							
			DWC		DNC		PWC		PNC	
			Pre-period	Post-period	Pre-period	Post-period	Pre-period	Post-period	Pre-period	Post-period
0	Screen score	M	30.44		27.32		29.87		27.42	
		V	132.94		90.82		158.51		139.24	
		n	49		56		47		57	
0–2	Total score	M	85.83	59.59	80.23	66.74	86.52	60.61	82.02	66.73
		V	458.90	606.29	373.33	638.32	703.58	1122.6	613.37	879.50
		n	42	42	47	47	42	42	46	46
0–6	Total score	M	85.94	41.51	79.50	49.13	87.18	34.78	81.40	55.17
		V	472.57	392.59	377.75	804.98	703.91	379.68	542.09	1241.6
		n	35	35	44	44	33	33	40	40
0–12	Total score	M	35.33	35.42	77.16	38.96	84.72	28.31	78.51	39.86
		V	475.07	737.21	328.54	371.10	695.10	738.49	568.18	855.40
		n	33	33	30	30	29	29	29	29
2–6	Total score	M	60.45	41.51	65.27	49.13	58.45	34.78	64.55	55.17
		V	583.56	392.59	642.24	804.98	1081.0	379.68	813.40	1241.6
		n	35	35	44	44	33	33	40	40
6–12	Total score	M	41.45	35.42	36.80	38.96	34.24	28.31	44.44	39.86
		V	382.85	737.21	200.03	371.10	392.32	738.49	857.01	855.50
		n	33	33	30	30	29	29	29	29

M, mean; *V*, variance

Table 14b. Screening scores, comparing combined counselling versus no counselling and combined drug versus placebo treatments: Bombay

	Counselling	No counselling	Drug	Placebo
Mean	30.2	27.4	28.8	28.5
SD	12.00	10.69	10.58	12.17

assessment of reliability were carried out during meetings of investigators held in Copenhagen and London. It was confirmed that a score of over 11 points on the GHQ served to identify correctly a psychiatric case. A validation study was carried out using total scores on the PSE and the GHQ. In all, 60 subjects (30 out-patients and 30 relatives in the waiting room as controls) were included in the study at each centre; results showed the Pearson correlation coefficients between the GHQ and PSE scores as follows: 0.94 for Bombay, 0.88 for Ibadan, 0.80 for London and 0.82 for Tokyo.

There was very little overlap in any of the centres between the screening scores of patients (over 11) and scores of accompanying relatives who acted as controls

Table 15a. Screening and total scores, General Health Questionnaire: Ibadan

Period			Treatment group							
			DWC		DNC		PWC		PNC	
			Pre-period	Post-period	Pre-period	Post-period	Pre-period	Post-period	Pre-period	Post-period
0	Screen score	M	23.01		23.50		22.42		22.15	
		V	86.49		87.98		58.52		57.00	
		n	52		48		47		51	
0–2	Total score	M	76.04	53.56	78.65	54.56	72.23	59.16	73.90	58.00
		V	279.41	289.29	261.14	342.64	188.18	333.85	198.88	306.84
		n	48	48	46	46	42	42	43	43
0–6	Total score	M	74.17	45.40	78.58	42.86	72.39	44.00	74.35	46.64
		V	268.00	223.04	276.62	284.31	188.87	353.84	199.80	274.23
		n	40	40	43	43	38	38	37	37
0–12	Total score	M	73.89	35.17	79.60	37.70	72.18	37.93	75.06	38.31
		V	271.89	355.48	279.14	378.81	203.96	306.06	201.61	344.09
		n	39	39	40	40	32	32	32	32
2–6	Total score	M	52.15	45.40	53.83	42.86	59.44	44.00	57.16	46.64
		V	274.38	223.04	345.72	284.31	311.09	353.84	322.51	274.23
		n	40	40	43	43	38	38	37	37
6–12	Total score	M	45.15	35.17	42.62	37.70	41.78	37.93	46.28	38.31
		V	226.34	355.48	281.38	378.81	339.80	306.06	271.26	344.09
		n	39	39	40	40	32	32	32	32

M, mean; *V*, variance

Table 15b. Screening scores, comparing combined counselling versus no counselling and combined drug versus placebo treatments: Ibadan

	Counselling	No counselling	Drug	Placebo
Mean	22.7	22.8	23.3	22.3
SD	8.52	8.47	9.29	7.56

(under 11), thus corroborating the efficacy of the GHQ (with cut-off score of about 11) in distinguishing between patients and non-patients. It has been reported (Newson-Smith and Hirsch 1979) in a study of patients just admitted following overdose, that patients with GHQ scores over 20 are generally unlikely to remit spontaneously over the next month while those who score under 20 remit spontaneously at a much higher rate.

The validity of these scales in this investigation was amply demonstrated by the changes in scores over time, consistently showing differences between treatment groups, and by satisfactory between-measures reliability. Correlations between GHQ and PSE total scores at baseline were 0.47 in London, 0.56 in

Table 16a. Screening and total scores, General Health Questionnaire: London

Period			Treatment group							
			DWC		DNC		PWC		PNC	
			Pre-period	Post-period	Pre-period	Post-period	Pre-period	Post-period	Pre-period	Post-period
0	Screen score	M	29.56		30.53		28.65		29.05	
		V	131.33		143.04		125.66		121.88	
		n	41		45		41		38	
0–2	Total score	M	87.18	69.26	88.81	69.67	83.61	66.95	86.94	72.13
		V	669.20	1066.5	522.38	787.34	527.02	579.80	635.44	796.56
		n	38	38	43	43	41	41	36	36
0–6	Total score	M	86.97	51.32	88.81	58.02	83.61	50.61	86.94	64.30
		V	685.59	800.98	522.38	790.77	527.02	607.65	635.44	824.99
		n	37	37	43	43	41	41	36	36
0–12	Total score	M	85.45	41.66	89.94	48.47	81.82	38.48	84.25	57.45
		V	665.91	298.06	508.93	784.01	518.63	528.94	572.49	616.45
		n	24	24	34	34	29	29	20	20
2–6	Total score	M	67.64	51.32	69.97	58.02	66.95	50.61	72.13	64.30
		V	996.28	800.98	787.34	790.77	579.80	607.65	796.56	824.49
		n	37	37	43	43	41	41	36	36
6–12	Total score	M	52.54	41.66	56.88	48.47	46.69	38.48	62.15	57.45
		V	814.66	298.06	959.81	784.01	619.73	528.94	777.13	616.45
		n	24	24	34	34	29	29	20	20

M, mean; *V*, variance

Table 16b. Screening scores, comparing combined counselling versus no counselling and combined drug versus placebo treatments: London

	Counselling	No counselling	Drug	Placebo
Mean	29.1	29.9	30.1	28.8
SD	11.17	11.50	11.66	11.06

Bombay, 0.16 in Ibadan and 0.54 in Tokyo. At week 6 the corresponding correlations were 0.63, 0.77, 0.29 and 0.61. Ibadan stands out for its low correlations. Combining all centres, the correlation at week 0 was 0.42, and that at week 6 was 0.61.

5.2 Overall Comparisons Among Centres

In a multicentre trial in which the centres may be very different, it is obviously useful to examine the results from each centre separately; nevertheless, conclu-

Table 17 a. Screening and total scores, General Health Questionnaire: Tokyo

Period			Treatment group							
			DWC		DNC		PWC		PNC	
			Pre-period	Post-period	Pre-period	Post-period	Pre-period	Post-period	Pre-period	Post-period
0	Screen score	M	34.16		27.60		35.00		20.70	
		V	263.74		163.33		125.44		69.06	
		n	6		15		7		17	
0–2	Total score	M	97.33	79.66	82.76	61.84	97.14	69.71	71.20	63.00
		V	757.22	867.56	581.25	547.51	532.69	554.20	338.56	417.20
		n	6	6	13	13	7	7	10	10
0–6	Total score	M	97.33	74.33	82.76	55.69	97.14	73.85	82.50	63.33
		V	757.22	574.22	581.25	728.67	532.69	482.69	213.58	109.56
		n	6	6	13	13	7	7	6	6
0–12	Total score	M								
		V				(Cells too small)				
		n								
2–6	Total score	M	79.66	74.33	61.84	55.69	69.71	73.85	66.83	63.33
		V	867.56	574.22	547.51	728.67	554.20	482.69	610.47	109.56
		n	6	6	13	13	7	7	6	6
6–12	Total score	M								
		V				(Cells too small)				
		n								

M, mean; *V*, variance

Table 17 b. Screening scores, comparing combined counselling versus no counselling and combined drug versus placebo treatments: Tokyo

	Counselling	No counselling	Drug	Placebo
Mean	34.6	23.9	29.5	24.9
SD	13.14	11.03	17.77	11.17

sions must ultimately be related to the results of an overall analysis of the complete design. This requires a multifactorial analysis of variance in which the two types of treatment constitute two factors, the centres a third, and the assessments at different intervals a fourth. The fourth of these implies a model based on repeated measurements. In this analysis the effects of treatment appear as interactions with time, i.e. between first and last assessments.

Because there were so few cases in the Tokyo centre, it was omitted from the following analysis.

5.2.1 Comparison of GHQ Total Scores at the Start of the Trial

The mean scores of 514 patients in the centres were: Bombay 81.83, London 87.13 and Ibadan 76.60. The overall test shows that these differences are very highly significant ($F_{(2,502)}=14{,}85$; $p<0.001$). The Bombay mean falls midway between that of London and that of Ibadan; the latter centre was 'mildest' of the three. From the clinical point of view, however, these differences are negligible.

In the following analyses the results described were adjusted for the initial differences in starting points. Table 18 is given in full to serve as an example of the overall analyses of variance.

5.2.2 Comparison of GHQ Scores Between Weeks 0 and 2

For the total of 514 patients the mean score at week 0 was 81.85; at Week 2 the mean had fallen to 63.18 – an improvement of 18.67 points, or 22.81% of the initial score. This is very highly significant ($F_{(1,502)}=335{,}50$; $p<0.001$). None of the other differences achieved statistical significance, which signifies that this improvement was unrelated to the treatments given (Tables 19 and 20).

5.2.3 Comparison of GHQ Scores Between Weeks 0 and 6

For the comparison of GHQ scores between weeks 0 and 6, the number of cases had fallen by 47 from 514 to 467, a loss of 9.14%. The mean score decreased by 33.01 points from 81.66 to 48.65, or 40.42%. Not surprisingly, this is very highly significant ($p<0.001$).

Table 18. Analysis of variance summary table: General Health Questionnaire total scores, weeks 0–6; combined Bombay, Ibadan, London

Source	df	Sum of squares	Mean squares	F	p
Drug (A)	1	1.12492	1.12492		
Counselling (B)	1	3681.66	3681.66	5.179	0.022
AB	1	978.383	978.383	1.376	0.240
Centre (C)	2	20833.6	10416.8	14.653	<0.001
AC	2	91.7781	45.8891		
BC	2	880.777	440.388		
ABC	2	276.312	138.156		
Between-group error	455	323462.0	710.906		
Period (D)	1	252504.0	252504.0	725.134	<0.001
AD	1	380.344	380.344	1.092	0.297
BD	1	3895.92	3895.92	11.188	0.001
ABD	1	1025.77	1025.77	2.946	0.083
CD	2	3317.17	1658.58	4.763	0.009
ACD	2	594.201	297.101		
BCD	2	5227.63	2613.82	7.506	<0.001
ABCD	2	109.567	54.7835		
Witin-group error	455	158439.0	348.217		

Table 19. General Health Questionnaire total score: means, variances, and percent change; combined Bombay, Ibadan, London

Period		Treatment group							
		DWC		DNC		PWC		PNC	
		Pre-period	Post-period	Pre-period	Post-period	Pre-period	Post-period	Pre-period	Post-period
0–2	M	83.1	60.9	82.6	63.8	80.8	62.2	80.9	65.7
	V	479.82	665.07	401.89	628.11	510.72	690.87	504.88	691.18
	C	26.7%		22.8%		23.0%		18.8%	
0–6	M	82.4	46.1	82.3	50.0	81.1	43.1	80.9	55.4
	V	504.81	482.71	413.4	666.46	503.27	495.28	485.52	842.31
	C	44.1%		39.2%		46.9%		31.5%	
0–12	M	81.6	37.4	82.1	41.7	79.6	34.9	79.3	45.2
	V	472.08	479.98	396.55	532.34	493.13	538.61	437.28	657.85
	C	54.2%		49.2%		56.2%		43.0%	
2–6	M	60.1	46.1	62.9	50.0	61.6	43.1	64.6	55.4
	V	650.87	482.71	636.4	666.46	651.18	495.28	683.52	842.3
	C	23.3%		20.5%		30.0%		14.2%	
6–12	M	46.4	37.4	45.4	41.7	40.9	34.9	50.9	45.2
	V	445.24	479.98	547.07	532.34	472.28	538.61	658.62	657.85
	C	19.4%		8.1%		14.7%		11.2%	

M, mean; *V*, variance; *C*, percent change

By the 6th week, taking all centres together, counselling had shown its superiority to no counselling very clearly ($p < 0.001$; see Tables 18–20), but an equally significant interaction between counselling and centres showed that this was not true for all the centres. In Bombay and London, counselled patients improved by 44.4 and 34.3 points, respectively, compared with 30.4 and 26.7 for the controls, an advantage of 14.0 points in Bombay but only 7.6 points in London. In Ibadan the corresponding improvements were by 28.6 and 31.7 points.

Examining the data for a possible interaction between drugs and counselling reveals no significant effect. Thus, counselling was not significantly affected regardless of whether or not the patient received drug, nor was the efficacy of drug treatment significantly affected whether the patient received counselling or not.

5.2.4 Comparison of GHQ Scores Between Weeks 6 and 12

The changes that occurred between weeks 6 and 12 must be considered against their background. In fact, all groups of patients continued to improve, their mean score falling by 6.11 points from 45.92 to 39.81, i.e. an improvement of 13.3% over the score at week 6. This is very highly significant ($F_{(1,359)} = 32.81$; $p < 0.001$). None of the other *F* ratios was significant. However, the effects of the various treatments maintained to some extent their relative positions during the last 6 weeks. Hence, when the comparisons are made between weeks 0 and 12, the

Table 20. General Health Questionnaire total scores for periods 0–2 and 0–6; contrasts of whether amount of improvement on drug was different from that on placebo and whether amount of improvement on counselling was different from that on non-counselling

Centre	Treat-ment	Period 0–2			Period 0–6		
		Week 0	Week 2	*p*	Week 0	Week 6	*p*
Bombay	D	83.0	63.1	NS	82.7	45.3	NS
	P	84.3	63.7		84.3	45.0	
	C	86.2	60.1	0.003	85.9	41.5	0.001
	NC	81.1	66.7		79.5	49.1	
Ibadan	D	77.3	54.1	0.001	76.4	44.1	NS
	P	73.1	58.6		73.3	45.3	
	C	74.1	56.4	NS	73.3	44.7	NS
	NC	76.3	56.3		76.5	44.8	
London	D	88.0	69.5	NS	87.9	54.7	NS
	P	85.3	69.5		85.3	57.5	
	C	85.4	68.1	NS	85.3	51.0	NS
	NC	87.9	70.9		87.9	61.2	
Tokyo	D	90.1	70.8	NS	90.1	65.0	NS
	P	84.2	66.4		89.8	68.6	
	C	97.2	74.7	NS	97.2	74.1	NS
	NC	77.0	62.4		82.6	59.5	
All centres	D	82.8	62.4	NS	82.3	48.0	NS
	P	80.9	63.7		81.0	49.3	
	C	82.0	61.6	NS	81.7	44.6	0.001
	NC	81.8	64.8		81.6	52.7	

D, drug; *P*, placebo; *C*, counselling; *NC*, non-counselling

general improvement from 80.6 to 39.8 (50.6%) is highly significant ($F_{(1,359)}=910.69$; $p<0.001$) (Tables 19 and 21).

Counselling versus no counselling was also advantageous ($F_{(1,359)}=7.00$; $p=0.008$), but it would not be unreasonable to say that it was not uniform among the centres, i.e. the interaction between counselling treatment and centres is just significant ($F_{(2,359)}=3.72$; $p=0.025$). Table 21 shows that counselling was associated with greater improvement than no counselling in London (decrease with counselling, 43.5; with no counselling, 33.9) and in Bombay (decrease with counselling, 53.1; with no counselling, 38.4) but not in Ibadan (decrease with counselling, 35.4; with no-counselling, 39.3) (see Fig. 2).

Table 21. General Health Questionnaire total scores for periods 0–12 and 6–12; contrasts of whether amount of improvement on drug was different from that on placebo and whether amount of improvement on counselling was different from that on non-counselling

Centre	Treat-ment	Period 0–12			Period 6–12		
		Week 0	Week 12	p	Week 6	Week 12	p
Bombay	D	81.3	37.2	NS	39.1	37.1	NS
	P	81.6	34.1		39.3	34.1	
	C	85.0	31.9	0.006	37.8	31.9	NS
	NC	77.8	39.4		40.6	39.4	
Ibadan	D	75.7	36.4	NS	43.9	36.4	NS
	P	73.6	38.1		44.0	38.1	
	C	73.0	37.6	NS	43.5	36.6	NS
	NC	77.3	38.0		44.5	38.0	
London	D	87.6	45.1	NS	54.7	45.1	NS
	P	83.0	48.0		54.4	48.0	
	C	83.6	40.1	NS	49.6	40.1	NS
	NC	86.9	53.0		59.5	53.0	
All centres	D	81.9	39.6	NS	45.9	39.6	NS
	P	79.4	40.1		45.9	40.1	
	C	80.6	36.2	0.008	43.6	36.2	NS
	NC	80.7	43.5		48.2	43.5	

D, drug; *P*, placebo; *C*, counselling; *NC*, non-counselling

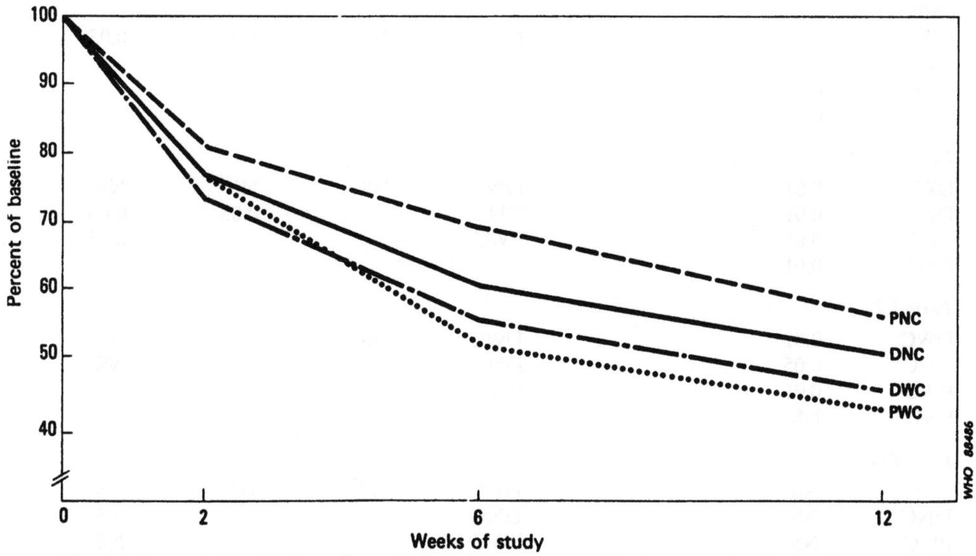

Fig. 2. General Health Questionnaire total scores at weeks 0, 2, 6, 12; *DWC*, diazepem with counselling; *DNC*, diazepam with no counselling; *PWC*, placebo with counselling; *PNC*, placebo with no counselling

5.3 Within-Centre Comparisons (Between Methods and Treatment)

Assessments were made with the GHQ at the start of the trial (week 0) and after 2, 6 and 12 weeks, however not at all centres. The formal end of the trial was at 6 weeks, but the physician could continue treatment if this was thought advisable.

Total scores on the GHQ were analysed by comparing the changes in scores among all the four types of treatment: drug with counselling (DWC), drug with no counselling (DNC), placebo with counselling (PWC) and with no counselling (PNC) (see Tables 14–17, 20–25). In addition, the effects of the main treatments (drugs and counselling) are reported here. The accompanying tables show that the analysis dealt with all possible intervals, but only the main ones, those from weeks 0 to 2 and from weeks 0 to 6, are described in detail here. The analyses described here compare only two treatments and therefore use t-tests.

Table 22. Post hoc analyses of pre- to post-period change within treatments and comparisons of amount of change between treatments (General Health Questionnaire total scores): Bombay

Within treatments: comparison of pre- to post-period		Between treatments: comparison of amount of change			
			DNC	PWC	PNC
Period 0–2					
DWC	0.01	DWC	NS	NS	NS
DNC	0.01	DNC		NS	NS
PWC	0.01	PWC			NS
PNC	0.01				
Period 0–6					
DWC	0.01	DWC	NS	NS	0.05
DNC	0.01	DNC		0.01	NS
PWC	0.01	PWC			
PNC	0.01				
Period 0–12					
DWC	0.01	DWC	NS	NS	NS
DNC	0.01	DNC		0.05	0.05
PWC	0.01	PWC			0.05
PNC	0.01				
Period 2–6					
DWC	0.01	DWC	NS	NS	NS
DNC	0.05	DNC		NS	NS
PWC	0.01	PWC			NS
PNC	NS				
Period 6–12					
DWC	NS	DWC	NS	NS	NS
DNC	NS	DNC		NS	NS
PWC	NS	PWC			NS
PNC	NS				

Figures are values for $p(\leqq)$.

Table 23. Post hoc analyses of pre- to post-period change within treatments and comparisons of amount of change between treatments (General Health Questionnaire total scores): Ibadan

Within treatments: comparison of pre- to post-period		Between treatments: comparison of amount of change	DNC	PWC	PNC
Period 0–2					
DWC	0.01	DWC	NS	NS	NS
DNC	0.01	DNC		0.05	NS
PWC	0.01	PWC			NS
PNC	0.01				
Period 0–6					
DWC	0.01	DWC	NS	NS	NS
DNC	0.01	DNC		NS	NS
PWC	0.01	PWC			NS
PNC	0.01				
Period 0–12					
DWC	0.01	DWC	NS	NS	NS
DNC	0.01	DNC		NS	NS
PWC	0.01	PWC			NS
PNC	0.01				
Period 2–6					
DWC	NS	DWC	NS	NS	NS
DNC	0.01	DNC		NS	NS
PWC	0.01	PWC			NS
PNC	0.01				
Period 6–12					
DWC	0.05	DWC	NS	NS	NS
DNC	NS	DNC		NS	NS
PWC	NS	PWC			NS
PNC	NS				

Figures are values for $p(\leqq)$.

5.3.1 Comparisons on Total GHQ Scores Between Weeks 0, 2 and 6

In the comparisons between weeks 0 and 2, weeks 0 and 6, and weeks 0 and 12, the mean scores at week 0 differ because the drop-outs between weeks 2 and 6 not only diminish the number of cases but also alter the values of the week 0 mean scores.

5.3.1.1 Bombay

Analysis of the Screening Score did not indicate differences among the treatments at the Bombay centre. At the start of the trial there were no significant differences in total GHQ scores among the four treatment groups. In the next 2 weeks all treatment groups together improved from a mean of 83.52 to 63.59, a decrease (improvement) of 19.93 points, which is very highly significant statistically

Table 24. Post hoc analyses of pre- to post-period change within treatments and comparisons of amount of change between treatments (General Health Questionnaire total scores): London

Within treatments: comparison of pre- to post-period		Between treatments: comparisons of amount of change			
			DNC	PWC	PNC
Period 0–2					
DWC	0.01	DWC	NS	NS	NS
DNC	0.01	DNC		NS	NS
PWC	0.01	PWC			NS
PNC	0.01				
Period 0–6					
DWC	0.01	DWC	NS	NS	NS
DNC	0.01	DNC		NS	NS
PWC	0.01	PWC			NS
PNC	0.01				
Period 0–12					
DWC	0.01	DWC	NS	NS	NS
DNC	0.01	DNC		NS	NS
PWC	0.01	PWC			NS
PNC	0.01				
Period 2–6					
DWC	0.05	DWC	NS	NS	NS
DNC	NS	DNC		NS	NS
PWC	0.05	PWC			NS
PNC	NS				
Period 6–12					
DWC	NS	DWC	NS	NS	NS
DNC	NS	DNC		NS	NS
PWC	NS	PWC			NS
PNC	NS				

Figures are values for $p(\leqq)$.

($p < 0.001$). However, no differences in improvement were to be found among the four treatment groups (see Tables 14 and 22). Drug and placebo groups decreased 19.9 and 20.6, respectively. Adding together the scores on drug and placebo sub-groups, the score of the counselling group fell from 86.2 to 60.1 (26.1 points) and that of the no-counselling group from 81.1 to 66.7 (14.4 points). However, the two groups did not differ significantly at the end of the 2nd week, i.e. the amount of improvement in the counselled group was significantly greater than that in the controls ($t = 3.01$; $p < 0.01$).

Further improvement occurred in all treatment groups, and by week 6 this was highly significant, but now differences in the respective states of the treatment groups appeared. The means of counselling and no counselling groups had fallen to 38.34 and 52.01, respectively; the difference of 13.76 was very highly significant (SE for the 68 and the 84 cases; 4.21; $t = 3.27$; $p < 0.001$). In contrast, means of drug

Table 25. Post hoc analyses of pre- to post-period change within treatments and comparisons of amount of change between treatments (General Health Questionnaire total scores): Tokyo

Within treatments: comparison of pre- to post-period		Between treatments: comparisons of amount of change			
			DNC	PWC	PNC
Period 0–2					
DWC	NS	DWC	NS	NS	NS
DNC	NS	DNC		NS	NS
PWC	0.05	PWC			NS
PNC	NS				
Period 0–6					
DWC	NS	DWC	NS	NS	NS
DNC	0.05	DNC		NS	NS
PWC	NS	PWC			NS
PNC	NS				
Period 2–6					
DWC	NS	DWC	NS	NS	NS
DNC	NS	DNC		NS	NS
PWC	NS	PWC			NS
PNC	NS				

Figures are values for $p(\leqq)$.

and placebo groups had fallen to 45.75 and 45.95, respectively. Examination of the details shows the obvious superiority of placebo with counselling over placebo with no counselling and over drugs with no counselling.

5.3.1.2 Ibadan

The results at the Ibadan centre (Tables 15 and 23) can be described very quickly. Analysis of the Screening Score did not indicate differences among the treatment groups. Although all treatment groups had improved considerably at week 2, and even more so at week 6, only one significant difference appeared temporarily among the various treatments. This was a highly significant advantage of drugs ($p < 0.001$) over placebo by week 2. This effect had faded by week 6, however. The group means are as follows: drug and placebo, 54.05 and 58.57 at week 2, and 44.08 and 45.30 at week 6, respectively; counselling and no counselling, 56.17 and 56.22 at week 2, and 44.72 and 44.61 at week 6, respectively.

5.3.1.3 London

The results at the London centre (Tables 16 and 24) were similar to those in Bombay and Ibadan. Analysis of the Screening Score did not indicate differences among the treatment groups. The improvement in all treatment groups was very highly significant by week 2 and by week 6. In the last 4 weeks the improvement was almost as great as in the first 2. Tests of significance appear to suggest that the improvement was much less here, but this is because the variability of results had become greater by the 6th week. Although statistical tests among the four treatment groups show non-significant differences, the difference between counselling (50.95) and no counselling (60.88) at week 6 is significant (SE for the 78 and the 79 cases, 4.38; $t = 2.27$; $p < 0.02$ and $p < 0.03$, respectively). In view of the many tests being made, this result must be accepted with great caution.

5.3.1.4 Tokyo

The small numbers of cases seen at the Tokyo centre (Tables 17 and 25) made it difficult to carry out complete analyses. Furthermore, the statistical test of Screening Scores showed that the groups differed significantly, results which were paralleled by the initial GHQ scores. These were, for Screening and GHQ, respectively: drug with counselling, 34.16 and 97.33; drug with no counselling, 27.60 and 82.76; placebo with counselling, 35.00 and 97.14; and placebo and no counselling, 20.70 and 71.20. Although all treatment groups showed improvement by weeks 2 and 6, not surprisingly, none of the differences examined reached statistical significance.

5.3.1.5 Summary

It can be concluded that, within each centre, all groups of patients benefited (as measured by total score on the GHQ) from participation in the trial. This improvement showed itself quickly even by the 2nd week, and continued steadily until the 6th week. In addition, from the 2nd week counselling showed a significantly greater improvement than no-counselling, very obviously in Bombay and less so in London. There was a temporary advantage of drugs at week 2 in Ibadan. There were no differences among the results of treatments in Ibadan and Tokyo, but in the latter there were too few cases for results to be significant.

5.3.2 Comparisons on Total GHQ Scores Between Weeks 6 and 12

The option to continue the trial to week 12 was not taken up in Tokyo. Not surprisingly, the overall number of patients fell to 371 (a decrease of 27.8% from the original number in all centres together). These remaining patients are therefore a highly selected group from the original cohort, and it is therefore necessary to be cautious about drawing conclusions from them. One way of comparing the group of patients which received treatment for only 6 weeks and then left the trial, with the group which stayed on for 12 weeks is to examine the scores at week 0 for these two groups. This information can be obtained from Tables 14–17 and 20–25. For the 6-week group and the 12-week group, respectively, the scores are: drug with counselling, 90.3 and 80.7; drug with no counselling, 82.3 and 82.3; placebo with counselling, 87.1 and 79.3; and placebo with no counselling, 86.66 and 78.56. The group which terminated treatment at the end of 6 weeks had a slightly higher score on the initial GHQ than the group which stayed on.

The results in the individual centres show that all treatment groups continued to improve. It could also be argued that those patients who were dissatisfied with their treatment did not continue to attend, leaving in the trial those patients who had benefited from the treatments. To ascertain whether this was in fact the case, the mean score of all the patients who were assessed at week 6 can be compared with the corresponding score at week 6 of those patients who were assessed at week 12. For the 467 patients available at week 6, the mean scores were: drug with counselling, 46.1; drug with no counselling, 50.0; placebo with counselling 43.1; and placebo with no counselling, 55.4 (Table 19). The corresponding means for the 371 patients who stayed on for the full 12 weeks are: drug with counselling, 46.4; drug with no counselling, 45.4; placebo with counselling, 40.9; and placebo with no counselling, 50.9. Although the former figures are generally higher than the latter, it does not require statistical tests to show that the differences are indeed very small. Similarly an examination of the initial scores of the groups who did not complete 2 weeks or did not complete 6 weeks showed negligible differences at the beginning of the trial from the group which completed 12 weeks. It can be concluded that the continuing improvement from weeks 6 to 12 is not the result of a particular selection of patients.

In Bombay the further improvement in both counselling treatment groups was about the same, but the advantage of the counselled patients at 6 weeks was maintained to the 12th week.

5.4 GHQ Factor Scores, Weeks 0 to 2 to 6

Factor analysis of GHQ scores produces two factors which are of interest in the present study: factor B (anxiety and insomnia) consisting of items 14, 18, 39, 44, 45, 47 and 55 and factor C (social dysfunction) consisting of items 21, 22, 28, 30, 35, 36 and 42 (see Appendix B). In the following account, all centres are combined together.

5.4.1 GHQ Factor B (Anxiety and Insomnia)

Examination of the scores on factor B (Tables 26 and 27) showed that there were no significant differences between treatment groups at week 0. The mean score for counselling was 1.470 and that for no counselling was 1.471 (SE, 0.046; $t=-0.02$; NS); for drug it was 1.49 and for placebo 1.46 (SE, 0.046; $t=0.65$; NS). At the end of 2 weeks all scores had diminished (improved) at a highly significant level, but differences among the treatments had already appeared. Drug-treated patients had decreased their mean score to 1.05, a fall of 29.6% and those receiving placebo to 1.1 (26.5%), a difference in favour of drug treatment but not significantly so (SE, 0.050; $t=-1.00$; NS). Counselled patients had decreased their mean score to 1.0 (29.9% fall) and the non-counselled to 1.2 (9.7% fall), a highly significant advantage for the former (SE, 0.050; $t=-4.00$; $p<0.001$).

These changes continued until week 6. There was still no significant difference between drug treatment and placebo (means for both, 0.8; SE, 0.050), but counselling (mean 0.7) was obviously superior to no counselling (mean, 0.9; SE, 0.050; $t=-4.00$; $p<0.001$).

Table 26. General Health Questionnaire: factor B (anxiety/insomnia)

Period		DWC		DNC		PWC		PNC	
		Pre-period	Post-period	Pre-period	Post-period	Pre-period	Post-period	Pre-period	Post-period
0–2	M	1.48	1.00	1.49	1.10	1.46	1.06	1.45	1.12
	V	0.30	0.35	0.26	0.35	0.30	0.32	0.32	0.36
0–6	M	1.48	0.75	1.49	0.83	1.46	0.70	1.45	0.93
	V	0.30	0.29	0.26	0.32	0.30	0.28	0.32	0.37
0–12	M	1.48	0.63	1.49	0.78	1.46	0.65	1.45	0.87
	V	0.30	0.27	0.26	0.32	0.30	0.31	0.32	0.43
2–6	M	1.00	0.73	1.09	0.82	1.06	0.66	1.11	0.90
	V	0.35	0.27	0.35	0.31	0.29	0.23	0.36	0.36
6–12	M	0.73	0.56	0.72	0.64	0.59	0.52	0.79	0.70
	V	0.26	0.22	0.26	0.25	0.20	0.22	0.30	0.37

M, mean; *V*, variance

This continued further until week 12, despite the loss in number of cases from 503 to 371. From week 6 until week 12 the drug cases improved from 0.72 to 0.60 and the placebo cases from 0.68 to 0.61, but at the end of this period there was still no significant difference between the scores of the two groups (SE, 0.054; $t=-0.09$; NS). During this period counselling maintained its advantage (mean, 0.5) compared with no counselling (mean, 0.7), a difference which was still highly significant (SE, 0.053; $t=-3.77$; $p<0.01$).

5.4.2 GHQ Factor C (Social Dysfunction)

The results for factor C are quite similar to those for factor B, but on a smaller scale (Tables 28 and 29). At Week 0 group means were: drug, 1.53; placebo, 1.46 (SE, 0.038; $t=1.84$; NS); counselling, 1.52; no counselling, 1.48 (SE, 0.038; $t=1.05$; NS). By week 2 the drug-treated groups had decreased their mean score by a little more than had the placebo groups so that both now showed a mean of 1.3. For counselling and no counselling the means were also 1.3 (no difference). All groups had shown some improvement, but it was not statistically significant.

By week 6 further improvement had occurred, and this was now highly significant statistically. Again the difference between the drug groups was trivial (drug, 1.07; placebo, 1.08), but the mean for counselling had fallen to 1.0 and that for no counselling to 1.1 (SE, 0.044; $t=-2.27$; $p<0.05$). When so many statistical tests are being carried out on the same sample of patients, it is not prudent to draw conclusions from a probability level of $p<0.05$. The result for factor C can be said only to follow this general direction.

However, this trend was maintained during the next 6 weeks for the 371 patients who continued treatment. Again there was no significant difference between the drug (0.9) and placebo (0.9) groups, but counselling maintained its

Table 27. General Health Questionnaire: factor B (anxiety/insomnia); post hoc analyses of pre- to post-period change within treatments and comparison of amount of change between treatments

Within treatments: analysis of change		Between treatments: comparison of amount of change			
			DNC	PWC	PNC
Period 0–2					
DWC	0.01	DWC	NS	NS	NS
DNC	0.01	DNC		NS	NS
PWC	0.01	PWC			NS
PNC	0.01				
Period 0–6					
DWC	0.01	DWC	NS	NS	0.05
DNC	0.01	DNC		NS	NS
PWC	0.01	PWC			0.05
PNC	0.01				
Period 0–12					
DWC	0.01	DWC	NS	NS	0.01
DNC	0.01	DNC		NS	NS
PWC	0.01	PWC			0.05
PNC	0.01				
Period 2–6					
DWC	0.01	DWC	NS	0.01 [a]	0.05
DNC	0.01	DNC		0.01 [a]	0.05
PWC	0.01	PWC			0.01
PNC	0.05				
Period 6–12					
DWC	0.05	DWC	NS	NS	NS
DNC	NS	DNC		NS	NS
PWC	NS	PWC			NS
PNC	NS				

Figures are values for $p(\leq)$.
[a] PWC > DWC and DNC

superiority, with a mean of 0.8 in contrast to the no-counselling mean of 0.9 (SE, 0.0453; $t=2.21$; $p<0.05$).

5.5 Comparison of Scores on Present State Examination

The PSE was completed at weeks 0 and 6. Of course, it is rarely possible to give a patient an extensive psychiatric interview without it being revealed whether or not counselling had been experienced, but some attempt was made to prevent the assessor from knowing. In Bombay PSE assessment was carried out by the psychiatrist who had previously done the assignments to treatment, in Ibadan it was

Table 28. General Health Questionnaire: factor C (social dysfunction)

Period		DWC		DNC		PWC		PNC	
		Pre-period	Post-period	Pre-period	Post-period	Pre-period	Post-period	Pre-period	Post-period
0–2	M	1.55	1.27	1.51	1.26	1.48	1.28	1.45	1.25
	V	0.21	0.27	0.17	0.28	0.24	0.23	0.17	0.20
0–6	M	1.55	1.05	1.51	1.09	1.48	1.01	1.45	1.15
	V	0.21	0.21	0.17	0.27	0.24	0.21	0.17	0.25
0–12	M	1.55	0.54	1.51	1.04	1.48	0.98	1.45	1.06
	V	0.21	0.21	0.17	0.24	0.24	0.23	0.17	0.29
2–6	M	1.24	1.01	1.25	1.07	1.26	0.96	1.24	1.12
	V	0.28	0.19	0.28	0.26	0.23	0.21	0.20	0.25
6–12	M	0.99	0.86	0.97	0.92	0.93	0.82	1.05	0.93
	V	0.19	0.17	0.23	0.19	0.22	0.19	0.19	0.21

M, mean; *V*, variance

done by an investigator other than the counsellor, in Tokyo by a psychiatrist and in London by the counsellor.

As the PSE was designed to cover the full range of syndromes in psychiatry, only the first 40 items received any scores at baseline for the four centres. Even then there was considerable disparity among the centres as to which items were marked, and only items 1, 4, 5, 6, 7, 10, 11a, 35 and 36 (see Appendix B) had at least 20% responses in all centres. Moreover, the responses in each centre were not always distributed evenly among the treatments. Under these circumstances it is likely that syndrome scores will be sensitive to such inequalities, although total scores would be less so (Tables 30–35).

5.5.1 Comparison on PSE Total Scores Between Weeks 0 and 6

For the four centres the mean total scores on the PSE at week 0 were: Bombay, 16.7; Ibadan, 14.8; London, 19.0; and Tokyo, 31.5. The differences are highly significant, based on an analysis of variance for the centres at Bombay, Ibadan and London, and for all treatments.

In the three centres (excluding Tokyo, which had too few cases for an analysis of variance) there was a highly significant improvement over the scores at 6 weeks ($F_{(1,424)} = 585.48$; $p < 0.001$) regardless of treatments (see Tables 30 and 31). The same analysis showed that drug-treated cases, improving from 16.93 to 7.30 (a fall of 56.3%), was only just better than those with placebo, which improved from 16.86 to 8.73 (a fall of 48.3%) ($F_{(1,424)} = 4.22$; $p = 0.04$). The counselling group, which improved from 17.16 to 7.39 (56.9% fall), was significantly better than the no counselling group, which improved from 16.64 to 8.64 ($F_{(1,424)} = 5.82$; $p = 0.015$). Within the individual centres, the improvement was not significant in Tokyo (perhaps because of the few cases; see Tables 30 and 31). Although the

Table 29. General Heath Questionnaire: factor C (social dysfunction); post hoc analyses of pre- to post-period change within treatments and comparison of amount of change between treatments

Within treatments: analysis of change		Between treatments: comparisons of amount of change			
			DNC	PWC	PNC
Period 0–2					
DWC	NS	DWC	NS	NS	NS
DNC	NS	DNC		NS	NS
PWC	NS	PWC			NS
PNC	NS				
Period 0–6					
DWC	0.01	DWC	NS	NS	NS
DNC	0.01	DNC		NS	NS
PWC	0.01	PWC			0.01
PNC	0.01				
Period 0–12					
DWC	0.01	DWC	NS	NS	0.01
DNC	0.01	DNC		NS	NS
PWC	0.01	PWC			0.05
PNC	0.01				
Period 2–6					
DWC	0.01	DWC	NS	NS	NS
DNC	0.01	DNC		NS	NS
PWC	0.01	PWC			0.05
PNC	0.05				
Period 6–12					
DWC	0.05	DWC	NS	NS	NS
DNC	NS	DNC		NS	NS
PWC	NS	PWC			NS
PNC	NS				

Figures are values of $p(\leqq)$.

decrease in mean score was of the same order in all centres, it must be noted that the mean score in Tokyo was higher at week 6 than it was at week 0 in the other centres (see Table 30).

5.5.1.1 Bombay

At 6 weeks the mean total score for drug treatment at the Bombay centre had decreased from 16.58 to 7.26 and for placebo from 16.91 to 7.15. Neither at the beginning nor at the end were the differences significant (week 6: SE, 1.069; $t = 0.10$; NS). In contrast, whereas the mean with counselling had fallen from 16.98 to 5.45, that with no counselling had fallen from 16.55 to 8.63. The advantage of counselling can be regarded as statistically significant (SE, 1.048; $t = 3.03$; $p < 0.01$). See Tables 30 and 32.

Table 30a. Present State Examination: means, variances and percent change of total scores by treatment and centre

Centre		DWC		DNC		PWC		PNC	
		Week 0	Week 6	Week 0	Week 6	Week 0	Week 6	Week 0	Week 6
Bombay	M	16.82	5.34	16.386	8.79	17.15	5.57	16.72	8.45
	V	13.22	30.62	33.328	45.61	20.18	37.51	13.79	55.54
	C	68.3		46.32		67.49		49.50	
Ibadan	M	15.67	6.20	14.88	4.95	14.81	7.42	13.86	7.08
	V	26.31	22.91	16.56	21.62	33.09	30.45	19.03	24.50
	C	60.45		66.72		49.91		48.93	
London	M	20.31	9.31	17.51	9.35	18.16	10.66	20.43	13.20
	V	135.18	95.77	142.19	71.32	75.86	66.72	87.77	121.16
	C	54.96		46.63		41.30		35.39	
Tokyo	M	38.66	33.00	29.30	18.15	33.85	27.28	26.50	23.83
	V	142.89	523.67	55.44	157.05	61.26	87.34	56.58	59.13
	C	14.66		38.06		19.41		10.08	

M, mean; *V*, variance; *C*, percent change

Table 30b. Present State Examination: total scores by (drug) treatment, centre and week

	Bombay		Ibadan		London		Tokyo	
	Drug	Placebo	Drug	Placebo	Drug	Placebo	Drug	Placebo
Week 0	16.61	16.94	15.28	14.34	18.91	19.30	32.26	30.46
Week 6	7.07	7.01	5.58	7.25	9.25	11.93	22.84	25.69
Improvement	9.54	9.93	9.70	7.09	9.66	7.37	9.42	4.77
n	79	73	83	75	60	66	4	6

Table 31. Present State Examination: means, variances and percent change of total scores, combined centres: Bombay, Ibadan, London

	DWC		DNC		PWC		PNC	
	Pre-period	Post-period	Pre-period	Post-period	Pre-period	Post-period	Pre-period	Post-period
Mean	17.61	6.89	16.26	7.70	16.71	7.89	17.01	9.57
Variance	55.88	48.20	52.81	47.52	45.55	49.16	43.03	69.45
Percent change	60.87		52.64		52.78		43.74	

Pre- to post-period change

Group	$p (\leq)$
DWC	0.01
DNC	0.01
PWC	0.01
PNC	0.01

Comparison among treatments

	DNC	PWC	PNC
DWC	NS	NS	0.05
DNC		NS	NS
PWC			NS

Table 32. Present State Examination total scores for period 0–6; post hoc comparisons of relative change between treatments: Bombay

	DNC	PWC	PNC
DWC	0.05	NS	0.05
DNC		0.05[a]	NS
PWC			NS
Post hoc comparisons of pre- to post-period change			
DWC	0.01		
DNC	0.01		
PWC	0.01		
PNC	0.01		

Figures are values for $p(\leqq)$.
[a] PWC > DNC

Table 33. Present State Examination total scores for period 0–6; post hoc comparisons of relative change between treatments: Ibadan

	DNC	PWC	PNC
DWC	NS	NS	NS
DNC		NS	0.05
PWC			NS
Post hoc comparison of pre- to post-period change			
DWC	0.01		
DNC	0.01		
PWC	0.01		
PNC	0.01		

Figures are values for $p(\leqq)$.

5.5.1.2 Ibadan

Also at the Ibadan centre all treatments improved, but this centre has one finding which can be regarded as unusual. The score for the drug group fell from 15.26 to 5.55 and that for the placebo group from 14.34 to 7.25. There was an advantage of drug treatment (SE, 0.797; $t=2.13$; $p < 0.05$), but in view of the many statistical tests being carried out on the same sample of individuals, this advantage falls below an acceptable level of significance. See Tables 30 and 33.

5.5.1.3 London

All treatments at the London centre showed significant improvements, but none of the differences among them reached significant levels. For the sake of completeness, the significance tests at week 6 are given. Decreases in group means were: drugs from 18.86 to 9.33 and placebo from 19.19 to 11.81 (SE, 1.665; $t=1.49$; NS); counselling from 19.12 to 10.06 and no counselling from 18.95 to 11.24 (SE, 1.672; $t=0.71$; NS). See Tables 30 and 34.

Table 34. Present State Examination total scores for period 0–6; post hoc comparisons of relative change between treatments: London

	DNC	PWC	PNC
DWC	NS	NS	NS
DNC		NS	NS
PWC			NS
Post hoc comparisons of pre- to post-period change			
DWC	0.01		
DNC	0.01		
PWC	0.01		
PNC	0.01		

Figures are values for $p(\leqq)$.

Table 35. Present State Examination total scores for period 0–6; post hoc comparisons of relative change between treatments: Tokyo

	DNC	PWC	PNC
DWC	NS	NS	NS
DNC		NS	NS
PWC			NS
Post hoc comparisons of pre- to post-period change			
DWC	NS		
DNC	NS		
PWC	NS		
PNC	NS		

Figures are values for $p(\leqq)$.

5.5.1.4 Comment

The findings on the PSE and those on the GHQ are very much in accord, but although the differences in PSE scores may appear to be small, they indicate real clinical changes. For example, with GHQ scores the patients not receiving counselling improved by 35.3% over 6 weeks and those who did by 55.8%, an advantage of 20.5%. On the PSE scale the corresponding figures are 48.9% and 67.9%, an advantage for counselling of 19%.

5.5.2 Comparison of PSE Syndromal Scores (Weeks 0 to 6)

5.5.2.1 Syndrome Health, Worry and Tension

There was a highly significant improvement with all treatments, the mean score decreasing from 0.66 to 0.33 ($F_{(1,424)}=567.58$; $p<0.001$).

Table 36. Present State Examination syndrome 'autonomic anxiety', period 0–6, by treatment and centre

	Bombay		Ibadan		London	
	C	NC	C	NC	C	NC
Week 0	0.322	0.293	0.152	0.132	0.147	0.195
Week 6	0.048	0.112	0.065	0.048	0.084	0.099
Difference	0.274	0.181	0.087	0.084	0.063	0.096

C, counselling, *NC*, no counselling

5.5.2.2 Syndrome Autonomic Anxiety

In addition to the general overall improvement ($p < 0.001$), there were significant differences among the centres in the response to counselling ($F_{(2,423)} = 4.274$; $p = 0.014$).

From Table 36 it can be seen that initial scores in Bombay were higher than in the other two centres, the differences being very highly significant ($p < 0.001$). In Bombay the improvement among counselled patients was greater than among the non-counselled. In Ibadan it was about equal, and in London it was less.

5.5.2.3 Syndrome Thinking, Concentration

The usual general improvement also occurred ($p < 0.001$), but in addition there was a highly significant response to counselling. The means improved with counselling from 0.38 to 0.14 and with no counselling from 0.33 to 0.19 ($F_{(1,424)} = 11.06$; $p < 0.001$).

5.5.2.4 Syndrome Depressed Mood

The same applied to the scores on this syndrome. The counselling group improved from 0.31 to 0.15 and the no counselling from 0.24 to 0.16 ($F_{(1,424)} = 9.57$; $p = 0.003$).

5.5.2.5 Syndrome Self and Others

The usual general improvement also occurred ($p < 0.001$), but in addition there was a just significant response to the drug and counselling treatments. Those receiving drugs improved from 0.13 to 0.06 and those receiving placebo from 0.11 to 0.07 ($F_{(1,424)} = 4.02$; $p = 0.04$); those with counselling improved from 0.13 to 0.06 and those with no-counselling from 0.11 to 0.07 ($F_{(1,424)} = 4.26$; $p = 0.037$).

5.5.2.6 Syndrome Appetite, Sleep, Retardation and Libido

The usual general improvement also occurred ($p < 0.001$), but in addition there was a just significant response to the drug and counselling treatments. The drug group improved from 0.37 and 0.11 and the placebo group from 0.34 to 0.14

($F_{(1,423)}=5.28$; $p=0.021$); those with counselling improved from 0.38 to 0.11 and those without from 0.34 to 0.13 ($F_{(1,423)}=3.84$; $p=0.048$).

5.5.2.7 Syndrome Irritability

In addition to the usual general improvement for all treatments there was a significant improvement with counselling treatment. The mean for the counselling group improved from 0.55 to 0.22 and that for the no counselling group from 0.52 to 0.32 ($F_{(1,424)}=5.65$; $p=0.017$).

5.6 Treatment-Emergent Symptoms

The most common treatment-emergent symptoms are listed in Table 37. It can be seen here that their incidence is comparatively low, so much so that it is difficult

Table 37. Twenty-six treatment-emergent symptoms reported in total population, frequency of occurrence, combined across all centres and all treatments

Symptom	Time of first occurrence		Reported once/ more than once		Total
	Weeks 1–2	Weeks 3–6	Once	More than once	
Drowsiness	45 (7.3%)	13 (2.1%)	47 (7.6%)	11 (1.8%)	58 (9.4%)
Dryness of mouth	35 (5.7%)	14 (2.3%)	41 (6.6%)	8 (1.3%)	49 (7.9%)
Dizziness	31 (5.0%)	13 (2.1%)	38 (6.2%)	6 (1.0%)	44 (7.1%)
Physical tiredness	28 (4.5%)	11 (1.8%)	27 (4.4%)	12 (1.9%)	39 (6.3%)
Get up sudden, dizzy	29 (4.7%)	5 (0.8%)	30 (4.9%)	4 (0.6%)	34 (5.5%)
Interference with sexual function	8 (1.3%)	5 (0.8%)	11 (1.8%)	2 (0.3%)	13 (2.1%)
Non-specific somatic complication	5 (0.8%)	1 (0.2%)	5 (0.8%)	1 (0.2%)	6 (1.0%)
Headache	4 (0.6%)	1	4 (0.6%)	1	5 (0.8%)
Blurred vision	1 (0.2%)	1	2 (0.3%)	0	2 (0.3%)
Constipation	1	1	1 (0.2%)	1	2 (0.3%)
Aches, pains (non-specific)	1	0	1	0	1 (0.2%)
Anorexia	1	0	0	1	1
Anxious	0	1	1	0	1
Apathetic	0	1	1	0	1
Chest pains	1	0	1	0	1
Depression	1	0	0	1	1
Epigastric pain	1	0	0	1	1
Impatience	1	0	1	0	1
Menstrual irregularity	0	1	1	0	1
Nausea	0	1	1	0	1
Rapid pulse	0	1	1	0	1
Sleep disturbance	1	0	1	0	1
Sore throat	0	1	1	0	1
Taste disturbance	1	0	1	0	1
Weight gain	0	1	1	0	1
Withdrawn	1	0	1	0	1

Table 38. Time of first occurrence of ten most commonly reported treatment-emergent symptoms in the total population, combined across treatments

Symptom	Bombay		Ibadan		London		Tokyo	
Weeks	1–2	3–6	1–2	3–6	1–2	3–6	1–2	3–6
Drowsiness	11	5	14	5	11	2	9	1
Dryness of mouth	3	0	13	3	14	8	5	3
Dizziness	7	2	12	6	9	2	3	3
Physical tiredness	2	2	7	3	13	4	6	2
Get up sudden, dizzy	9	2	11	3	5	0	4	0
Interference with sexual function	1	0	4	1	3	3	0	1
Non-specific somatic complication	0	1	1	0	2	0	2	0
Headache	0	0	0	1	3	0	1	0
Blurred vision	0	1	1	0	0	0	0	0
Constipation	0	1	0	0	0	0	1	0

Figures are absolute numbers of patients.

Table 39. Time of first occurrence of ten most commonly reported treatment-emergent symptoms reported for each treatment, combined across centres, by treatment

Symptoms	DWC		DNC		PWC		PNC	
Weeks	1–2	3–6	1–2	3–6	1–2	3–6	1–2	3–6
Drowsiness	6	1	17	6	15	1	7	5
Dryness of mouth	8	6	14	2	7	2	6	4
Dizziness	7	2	11	3	8	5	5	3
Physical tiredness	8	3	6	1	7	5	7	2
Get up sudden, dizzy	10	1	5	2	8	2	6	0
Interference with sexual function	3	0	1	3	1	1	3	1
Non-specific somatic complication	1	0	2	0	1	1	1	0
Headache	2	0	1	0	0	0	1	1
Blurred vision	0	0	1	1	0	0	0	0
Constipation	0	0	0	0	1	0	0	1

Figures are absolute numbers of patients.

to carry out any statistical analysis on them. From Table 38 it can be seen that the incidence is approximately of the same order in all the centres, and Table 39 shows that this is also true for the four different combinations of treatment. It is particularly noteworthy that those patients who received neither drugs nor counselling had about the same incidence of treatment-emergent symptoms as those who received one or the other treatments or both. This was true even for 'drowsiness', the importance of which should not be underestimated. These results are in accord with clinical experience that treatment-emergent symptoms are of minor importance, when the doses are low, in the treatment and management of anxiety states and other neurotic conditions.

Some uncommon emergent symptoms appeared once only: anorexia, epigastric pain and menstrual irregularities in Bombay; sore throat, chest pains and disturbance of taste in Ibadan; non-specific aches and pains, rapid pulse, weight gain, nausea and 'appearing withdrawn' in London; and anxiety, impatience, depression, apathy and disturbance of sleep in Tokyo.

5.7 Physical Measurements

When the patients first entered the trial, a record was made of their weight, pulse rate, and systolic and diastolic blood pressures, both sitting and standing. Analysis of these variables under the influence of treatment and over the course of time shows that there were changes, but even though some of these were statistically significant ($p < 0.001$), the changes were quite trivial. For example, in Tokyo there was a decrease in the sitting diastolic blood pressure among those with counselling from 80.2 to 76.9 mm Hg and among those without counselling from 79.7 to 79.6 mm Hg ($p = 0.024$).

5.8 Brief Life Events Questionnaire

There were significant differences in the frequency of life events among the centres, with the most being reported in Bombay and London. There were no significant differences among treatment groups, either within the centres or in overall terms (see Table 40).

Using a count of the number of life events experienced, it was found that while there were no significant differences among the centres at week 6, a highly significant interaction ($p < 0.001$) between centres and counselling treatment appeared at week 12. There were more events associated with counselling than with no counselling in Bombay, Ibadan and London, but not in Tokyo. There were more associated with drug treatment than with placebo ($p < 0.001$), largely due to the group receiving drugs with counselling. This suggests that, not surprisingly, patients who were counselled gave much more information about themselves and their life experiences; on the other hand, however, the group with placebo and counselling had a low score.

The correlations between score on the BLEQ and that on the GHQ (representing severity of symptoms) were generally low, but significant at week 0; they were non-significant at weeks 6 and 12, except in London. GHQ total scores were significantly higher for those patients who had experienced one or more life events than for those who had not. Both methods of examining the data showed that more life stresses were associated with a greater severity of illness (symptoms) (see Table 41).

Table 40. Brief Life Events Questionnaire, weeks 6 and 12; number of items responded to per section, number and percent of subjects who responded per section, rank ordering of frequency of subjects responding

		Section						
		Illness/ injury	School	Work	Finance	Relation-ship	Child/ family	Other changes
London								
Week 6	I	72	7	63	32	66	31	21
($n = 156$)	S	59/38	7/4	55/35	26/17	53/34	25/16	21/13
	R	1	7	3	4	2	5	6
Week 12	I	46	3	35	13	26	16	7
($n = 103$)	S	34/33	3/3	31/30	11/11	24/23	13/13	7/7
	R	1	7	2	5	3	4	6
Bombay								
Week 6	I	54	21	59	47	30	32	71
($n = 152$)	S	46/30	21/14	49/32	43/28	25/16	29/19	60/39
	R	3	7	2	4	6	5	1
Week 12	I	42	21	52	42	22	29	55
($n = 120$)	S	35/29	21/18	43/36	39/33	19/16	27/23	47/39
	R	3.5	7	2	3.5	6	5	1
Ibadan								
Week 6	I	42	4	16	10	11	13	6
($n = 157$)	S	37/23	4/3	14/9	10/6	10/6	11/7	6/4
	R	1	7	2	5	4	3	6
Week 12	I	25	5	13	8	9	15	5
($n = 146$)	S	24/16	5/3	11/8	8/5	8/5	13/9	5/3
	R	1	6.5	3	5	4	2	6.5
Tokyo								
Week 6	I	8	3	8	2	5	1	3
($n = 32$)	S	7/22	3/9	7/22	2/6	4/13	1/3	3/9
	R	1.5	4.5	1.5	6	3	7	4.5
Week 12	I	2	2	4	0	0	0	0
($n = 16$)	S	2/13	2/13	3/19	0	0	0	0
	R	(not determined)						
Combined Centres								
Week 6	I	176	35	146	91	112	77	101
($n = 498$)	S	149/30	35/7	125/25	81/16	92/18	66/13	90/18
	R	1	7	2	5	3	6	4
Week 12	I	115	31	104	63	57	60	67
($n = 385$)	S	95/25	31/8	88/23	58/15	51/13	53/14	59/15
	R	1	7	2	4	6	5	3

I, number of items responded to per section; *S*, number/percentage of subjects responding per section; *R*, rank ordering of frequency of subjects responding

Table 41. Correlations between Brief Life Events Questionnaire (BLEQ) scores and General Health Questionnaire (GHQ) scores by centre and week

London		GHQ Week		
	Week	0	6	12
BLEQ	6	0.21	0.08	0.10
	12	0.21	0.11	0.13
Bombay		GHQ Week		
	Week	0	6	12
BLEQ	6	0.10	−0.03	0.11
	12	0.16	0.06	0.10
Ibadan		GHQ Week		
	Week	0	6	12
BLEQ	6	0.10	−0.04	−0.03
	12	0.05	0.03	0.05
Tokyo		GHQ Week		
	Week	0	6	12
BLEQ	6	0.06	0.08	0.21
	12	−0.03	0.12	0.06
All centres		GHQ Week		
	Week	0	6	12
BLEQ	6	0.19	0.04	0.06
	12	0.18	0.02	0.04

5.9 General Summary: Effects of Drugs and Counselling

This study set out to examine a number of questions requiring a complex design, and one would expect the answers to be correspondingly complex. In fact, however, there is a surprising consistency, even though not total, in the results reported.

The main assessment in the trial was with the GHQ, carried out at the start and at 2nd, 6th and 12th weeks. The overall analysis, i.e. for all centres simultaneously, showed that there was a steady and continuous improvement for all four treatment groups, clearly present at the 2nd week and continuing to the 12th week. At the 6th week a difference appeared among the treatments, and this showed that counselled patients did better than non-counselled. This difference was maintained to the 12th week. The results with the GHQ total score were seen also in regard to factor C (social dysfunction) although with a lower level of significance. Concerning factor B (anxiety and insomnia) scores, the results were the same as for total scores, with an additional slight advantage of drugs versus placebo at week 2, but a not statistically significant one. Tokyo was not included in this analysis because of the small number of patients seen there.

Results for the individual centres are similar. There was steady improvement in all treatment groups for the full length of the trial. By the 2nd week counselling showed an advantage over no counselling in Bombay, and this difference was still present by week 12.

The PSE was administered at the start of the trial and again at the 6th week. Its sensitivity is different from that of the GHQ because, in addition to showing that counselling (59.0% fall in scores) was better than no counselling (48.2% fall) ($p = 0.015$), it also showed that drug treatment (56.9% fall) was marginally better than placebo (48.1% fall) ($p = 0.038$). The discrepancy between the percentage fall and statistical tests of significance results from the tests, being applied to actual scores rather than to percentages.

Taking the centres separately, all showed the same general improvement with all four treatments. In addition, in Bombay the difference between counselling and no counselling and in Ibadan the difference between drugs and placebo reached a level of statistical significance.

The PSE yields seven syndromal subscores. All of these showed the same general improvement but differed among themselves in detail. 'Health, worry and tension' showed no differences among the four treatment groups, but counselling showed an advantage in regard to 'thinking and concentration', 'depressed mood', 'self and others', 'appetite, sleep, etc.' and 'irritability'. For 'autonomic anxiety' the same was true in Bombay, but this treatment and its control showed the same effect in Ibadan, and in London the counselled patients improved less. Finally, drug treatment was better than placebo for 'appetite, sleep, etc.' and marginally better for 'self and others'.

6 Results: Analysis of Counselling

In making comparisons among the centres, the data from Tokyo were omitted because of the small number of patients. Where relevant, the Tokyo results are reported.

6.1 Difference Among Centres in Amount of Counselling

6.1.1 Total Interview Time

It is obvious that the appointment system, whether half-hourly or hourly, largely determined the duration of the interviews. The mean duration of interviews was: in Bombay 28.0, in Ibadan 32.1 and in London 28.3 min. The variation is small, but the differences are statistically significant ($p = 0.013$). In Tokyo the duration was 51.6 min. For all the centres, the duration for patients receiving drug or placebo was 30.1 and 28.8 min, respectively (Table 42).

6.1.2 Number of Sessions of Counselling

In Bombay, Ibadan und London, the mean number of sessions was 4.9, 4.8 and 4.4, respectively; in the same order, the modal number was 6, 6 and 5. The figures for Tokyo were a mean of 2.6 and a mode of 2. In view of the fact that the duration of the sessions in Tokyo were about twice as long as that in the other centres, it can be concluded that the total time spent in counselling was about the same in all centres.

On none of these three variables was the difference between the patients receiving drugs and those receiving placebo statistically significant (Table 42).

6.2 Differences Among Centres in Methods of Counselling

Table 42 presents the full set of details on the percentage of time spent (averaged for each patient across all the sessions) on the eight different techniques, for the different centres and treatment groups. When centres are compared with regard to the amount of time spent on each of the counselling techniques, the differences are highly significant ($p < 0.001$, except for interpretation, where $p = 0.016$). There was no difference between drug and placebo groups. For convenience, Table 43 gives the data in summary form.

Table 42. Audit of Counselling part A by treatment and centre; interview time and method of counselling

		London		Bombay		Ibadan		Tokyo	
		DWC	PWC	DWC	PWC	DWC	PWC	DWC	PWC
Total interview time (min)	M	30.3	26.2	28.2	27.8	32.0	32.3	63.8	41.1
	V	64.166	44.205	66.421	66.469	225.78	150.94	499.48	658.92
	n	41	41	49	47	52	47	6	7
General conversation time (min)	M	0.5	0.7	2.2	3.1	22.2	22.5	26.9	15.3
	V	0.922	1.880	1.196	7.049	73.341	93.660	824.82	51.16
	n	41	41	49	47	52	47	6	7
Number of sessions	M	4.1	4.7	4.9	4.8	4.8	4.7	2.2	2.9
	Mode	5	5	6	6	6	6	2	2
Method of counselling (percent of time)									
History taking	M	10.2	10.3	16.0	18.6	22.9	23.4	30.0	27.5
	V	53.956	47.668	60.557	123.18	109.08	158.56	464.58	500.98
	n	41	41	49	47	52	47	6	7
Exploration	M	17.6	20.9	16.4	18.4	15.5	15.2	5.0	13.6
	V	137.91	206.43	48.491	96.534	80.552	80.002	68.75	83.67
	n	41	41	49	47	52	47	6	7
Permitting silence	M	2.4	0.8	2.3	1.8	5.8	6.2	2.1	2.7
	V	20.488	0.915	5.928	4.719	55.454	48.586	5.03	6.99
	n	41	41	49	47	52	47	6	7
Ventilation	M	45.7	45.3	32.6	27.6	8.2	8.5	2.9	12.7
	V	596.41	486.40	242.10	196.27	78.051	100.06	13.36	230.09
	n	41	41	49	47	52	47	6	7
Encouragement	M	5.2	6.1	13.8	12.5	13.4	12.5	8.3	14.5
	V	41.043	57.955	103.26	106.85	93.534	65.868	40.97	86.80
	n	41	41	49	47	52	47	6	7
Advice giving	M	4.0	2.7	5.8	4.7	21.6	21.5	27.5	21.1
	V	47.622	15.374	22.655	17.534	50.699	55.742	395.83	111.77
	n	41	41	49	47	52	47	6	7
Interpretation	M	8.3	7.9	7.6	9.1	10.8	10.9	9.0	8.0
	V	49.908	39.507	31.955	51.474	39.507	64.938	38.67	54.88
	n	41	41	49	47	41	47	6	7
Challenging	M	5.5	3.4	0.2	0.4	1.4	1.2	3.1	0
	V	31.339	13.543	0.564	2.533	7.434	9.480	13.4	0
	n	41	41	49	47	52	47	6	7

M, mean; *V*, variance

In spite of this, the order of importance of these techniques has a fair correspondence, the (rank-order) coefficient of concordance (W) being 0.69 and the probability of the null hypothesis being about 0.05 or less. In London 'ventilation' received 45.5% of the time and in Bombay 30.2%. Correspondingly, the figures for 'exploration' were 19.2% and 17.4%, and for 'history taking' they were 10.3% and 17.3%, giving the same rank ordering for these three variables. In Ibadan and

Table 43. Method of counselling: percent of time and rank ordering

	London		Bombay		Ibadan		Tokyo	
	%	rank	%	rank	%	rank	%	rank
History taking	10.3	3	17.3	3	23.2	1	28.7	1
Exploration	19.2	2	17.4	2	15.3	3	9.6	4
Permitting silence	1.6	8	2.1	7	6.0	7	2.4	7
Ventilation	45.5	1	30.1	1	8.3	6	8.2	6
Encouragement	5.7	5	13.2	4	13.0	4	11.6	3
Advice giving	3.4	7	5.3	6	21.5	2	24.1	2
Interpretation	8.1	4	8.3	5	10.9	5	8.5	5
Challenging	4.4	6	0.3	8	1.3	8	0.2	8

Tokyo 'history' and 'advice-giving' took the first two places with 23.1% and 21.5% and with 28.7% and 24.1% respectively. The greatest discrepancies in rank ordering were in regard to 'ventilation', which was given first place in London and Bombay but sixth in Ibadan and Tokyo, and in regard to 'advice giving', which came second in Ibadan and Tokyo but seventh and sixth in London and Bombay. In Ibadan third place was taken by 'exploration' (15.4%) and in Tokyo by 'encouragement' (11.6%). The techniques least used were 'permitting silence' and 'Challenging' (Table 43).

The time spent in 'general conversation' was also recorded, but in view of the fact that the instructions for recording had been interpreted differently, no analysis of these data was carried out.

6.3 Problem Areas Considered at Interview

There were 24 specified types of problems, in addition to 'other' (see Table 44). There was great similarity in the percentage of time spent on them in the different centres; the (rank-order) coefficient of concordance (W) for the whole set of 25 items was 0.799, which is very highly significant ($p<0.001$). In the total population the five problem areas upon which the greatest amount of time was spent were: illness/health, 29%; work, 12.5%; family relationships, 10.8%; money, 7.4%; and love/sexual relationships, 6.1%. It can be seen in Table 41 that differences between the amount of time occupied with problems relating to work were very highly significant statistically (error variance, 207.68; $p < 0.001$), the difference between the two highest, Bombay (17.50%) and London (11.9%) being very notable ($t=2.59$; df, 271; $p < 0.01$). The same applies to illness/health (error variance, 346.81; $p < 0.001$), in which Ibadan was the highest with 52.3%, followed by London with 18.9% ($t=9.12$; df, 257; $p < 0.001$).

For comparisons among centres and between drug treatments, the five problem areas with the most data were selected (see Table 45). The differences among centres on money, work and illness/health were very important ($p < 0.001$). There was no significant difference between drug and placebo among the five. Although

Table 44. Mean percent of time spent on interview problem areas

Problem area	Percent of total interview time				
	London	Bombay	Ibadan	Tokyo	Total
Money	1.2	6.2	14.6	1.5	7.4
Housing	3.1	2.7	0.5	3.3	2.1
Work	11.9	17.5	8.6	9.2	12.5
School/study	1.4	6.0	1.2	5.5	3.0
Legal problems	0.5	0.7	0.4	0	0.5
Child care	4.3	2.1	4.0	0.8	3.3
Loneliness	3.6	1.6	2.2	6.7	2.6
Illness/health	18.9	14.3	52.3	23.8	29.0
Bereavement	0.5	0.8	4.3	0.4	1.9
Pregnancy	0.8	0.3	2.0	0.2	1.0
Abortion	0.3	0.1	0.7	0	0.4
Family planning	0.8	1.3	0.2	0.6	0.8
Sexual problems	3.0	5.6	1.2	2.7	3.2
Love and sexual relationships	13.0	4.8	1.8	4.6	6.1
Family relationships	13.3	17.6	1.0	19.0	10.8
Social relationships	4.6	2.8	0.2	4.6	2.5
Divorce/separation	1.6	0	0.5	0.6	0.7
Gambling	0.5	0.1	0	0	0.2
Alcoholism	1.9	0.3	0	0.1	0.8
Religion	0.3	0.1	0	2.1	0.2
Racial/cultural	0.2	0	0	0	0.1
Drug abuse	0.0	0.1	0	0.2	0.1
Self doubt/lack of confidence	8.2	2.6	0.1	11.3	3.7
Abnormal fears or irrational thoughts	1.3	2.6	0.5	3.5	1.6
Other	4.8	9.0	3.2	0	5.4

Table 45. Audit of Counselling, time spent on problem areas, combined centres of London, Bombay, Ibadan

Problem area	Treatment	Mean	SD	*n*
Money	D	6.99	11.32	142
	P	8.52	12.67	135
Work	D	12.01	14.27	142
	P	13.37	15.39	135
Child care	D	3.13	8.99	142
	P	3.78	9.71	135
Loneliness	D	2.51	6.72	142
	P	2.23	4.56	135
Illness/health	D	25.94	25.08	134
	P	25.12	20.60	129
Family relationships [a]	D	14.84	15.41	71
	P	15.98	18.84	76

No differences were revealed between the two treatment groups for any of the five variables; *D*, drug; *P*, placebo.

[a] Excluding Ibadan, where most scores were zero.

there were no scores for family relationships in Ibadan, the results from this centre are included in Table 45 for completeness. To determine how similar the centres were in percentage of time spent on each problem area, a coefficient of concordance was calculated on the rank order of the 25 problem areas for three centres. The coefficient was highly significant ($W = +0.80$; $p < 0.001$), indicating a strong similarity in the rank order of problems covered among the centres. In the total population the five problem areas upon which the greatest amount of time was spent were: illness/health (29%), work (12.5%), family relationships (10.8%), money (7.4%) and love/sexual relationships (6.1%). Among the centres, considering only the first four ranks, illness/health came first in London, Ibadan and Tokyo but third in Bombay. Work came second in Bombay, third in Ibadan and fourth in London and Tokyo. Family relationships came first in Bombay and second in London and Tokyo.

These results can be summarized briefly with the simple statement that although there were differences in the absolute percentage of time spent in counselling on particular problem areas, there was still substantial similarity among the centres in the types of problems which received the greatest proportion of discussion.

6.4 Final Audit of Counselling

In the analyses for this section Tokyo was again excluded (although its data are recorded in Table 46). No significant differences were found between drug treatment groups.

6.4.1 Final Audit of Items

At the final session the counsellor rated the 25 items, on a five-point scale (0–4), for (a) the importance of the problem for the patient; (b) any identifiable progress (objective change) during counselling; and (c) the patient's change in feelings about the problem (subjective change). The results are shown in Table 46 and summarized in Table 47. Only nine of the items were analysed, owing to lack of data in some areas. These were: money, work, child care, loneliness, illness/health, bereavement, sex problems, love/sexual relationships and 'other'; for these the between-centre differences were very highly significant ($p < 0.001$). In the case of bereavement only the subjective change was significant ($p = 0.006$).

Excluding Tokyo with its mere four cases, it is evident that for almost all of these variables, the ratings for Bombay were higher than for the other centres. In general, subjective change rated higher than objective change.

A report on the Content of Counselling and its changes over time will appear as a separate publication.

Table 46. Final Audit of Counselling, importance, objective change, subjective change and overall evaluation of change, by treatment and centre

Item		London		Bombay		Ibadan		Tokyo	
		DWC	PWC	DWC	PWC	DWC	PWC	DWC	PWC
Money									
Imp	M	1.3	1.3	2.6	2.3	1.2	1.5	0.7	0.3
	V	0.69	0.20	0.44	0.72	1.40	1.25	1.33	0.33
	n	8	11	21	19	33	34	3	3
OC	M	0.5	0.0	2.5	2.0	0.9	0.9	0.0	0.7
	V	0.75	0.0	1.77	1.26	1.38	1.53	0.00	1.33
	n	8	11	21	19	28	30	3	3
SC	M	0.5	0.0	3.1	2.6	0.9	1.0	0.0	1.0
	V	0.75	0.00	0.31	0.55	1.45	1.63	0.00	3.00
	n	8	11	21	19	28	30	3	3
Work									
Imp	M	1.8	2.2	2.9	2.9	1.4	1.6	0.3	2.3
	V	0.81	0.94	0.62	0.87	1.78	1.91	0.25	4.33
	n	30	29	27	26	35	31	4	3
OC	M	1.2	1.6	2.9	3.0	1.3	1.2	0.0	2.0
	V	1.81	2.04	1.28	0.73	1.63	2.05	0.00	4.00
	n	30	29	27	26	28	25	4	3
SC	M	1.2	1.9	3.2	3.2	1.2	1.2	0.0	2.0
	V	1.89	2.12	0.69	0.59	1.67	2.02	0.00	4.00
	n	30	29	27	26	28	25	4	3
Child care									
Imp	M	2.0	2.2	3.0	2.3	1.0	1.0	1.0	0.5
	V	1.27	1.81	0.66	0.19	1.50	1.20	3.00	1.00
	n	11	12	6	4	26	20	3	4
OC	M	1.5	1.1	3.0	3.8	0.9	0.8	0.0	0.0
	V	1.52	1.24	0.00	0.19	1.73	2.03	0.00	0.00
	n	11	12	6	4	19	15	3	4
SC	M	1.7	1.6	3.0	3.5	0.9	0.7	0.7	0.0
	V	2.02	1.41	0.00	0.75	1.73	1.66	1.33	0.00
	n	11	12	6	4	19	15	3	4
Loneliness									
Imp	M	2.2	2.2	2.3	2.4	0.3	0.5	0.0	0.0
	V	1.01	0.26	0.22	0.23	0.54	1.01	0.00	0.00
	n	19	17	9	11	23	21	3	3
OC	M	1.2	1.3	3.0	2.8	0.5	0.7	0.0	0.0
	V	1.11	1.27	1.56	1.24	1.34	1.47	0.00	0.00
	n	19	17	9	11	11	11	3	3
SC	M	1.4	1.4	3.2	3.0	0.5	0.8	0.0	0.0
	V	1.18	1.41	0.62	1.27	1.34	1.79	0.00	0.00
	n	19	17	9	11	11	11	3	3

Table 46 (Continued)

Item		London		Bombay		Ibadan		Tokyo	
		DWC	PWC	DWC	PWC	DWC	PWC	DWC	PWC
Illness/health									
Imp	M	2.2	2.6	2.8	3.1	3.3	3.1	1.8	2.0
	V	1.18	0.54	0.40	0.24	0.60	0.54	1.58	2.67
	n	30	33	36	33	42	38	4	4
OC	M	2.3	2.8	3.6	3.5	2.6	2.7	1.8	1.0
	V	2.30	1.21	0.41	0.31	1.03	0.68	1.58	1.33
	n	29	33	36	33	43	38	4	4
SC	M	2.5	2.8	3.5	3.4	2.5	2.6	1.3	1.0
	V	2.18	0.89	0.47	0.66	1.23	0.71	2.25	1.33
	n	30	33	36	33	43	38	4	4
Bereavement									
Imp	M	1.0	1.0	1.2	1.8	0.4	0.8	0.0	0.0
	V	1.33	0.67	0.40	0.94	0.88	2.03	0.00	0.00
	n	6	3	9	8	22	18	3	3
OC	M	0.5	1.0	2.0	1.9	0.9	1.6	0.0	0.0
	V	1.25	2.00	3.33	3.61	1.65	2.73	0.00	0.00
	n	6	3	9	8	9	8	3	3
SC	M	0.8	1.0	2.7	3.1	0.9	1.9	0.0	0.0
	V	1.47	2.00	2.44	1.86	1.65	2.11	0.00	0.00
	n	6	3	9	8	9	8	3	3
Sexual problems									
Imp	M	1.8	1.6	3.3	3.4	0.3	0.5	2.0	0.0
	V	1.85	1.23	0.76	0.37	0.92	1.09	3.33	0.00
	n	12	8	16	14	23	19	4	3
OC	M	1.3	0.6	3.3	3.1	0.6	0.5	1.3	0.0
	V	2.06	1.23	1.19	1.27	1.14	1.05	2.25	0.00
	n	12	8	16	14	11	10	4	3
SC	M	1.5	0.9	3.3	3.3	0.6	0.5	1.5	0.0
	V	1.92	1.36	1.31	1.06	1.14	1.05	3.00	0.00
	n	12	8	16	14	11	10	4	3
Love/sexual relationships									
Imp	M	2.5	2.4	2.8	2.2	0.4	0.6	1.0	0.0
	V	0.73	0.94	0.64	1.14	0.94	1.39	4.00	0.00
	n	29	23	12	6	23	19	4	3
OC	M	0.9	1.6	2.9	1.8	0.8	0.8	0.5	0.0
	V	1.31	1.94	1.08	2.14	1.56	1.24	1.00	0.00
	n	29	26	12	6	10	11	4	3
SC	M	1.1	1.7	2.8	2.0	0.7	0.8	0.5	0.0
	V	1.50	1.74	1.14	2.33	1.47	1.24	1.00	0.00
	n	29	26	12	6	11	11	4	3

Table 46 (Continued)

Item		London		Bombay		Ibadan		Tokyo	
		DWC	PWC	DWC	PWC	DWC	PWC	DWC	PWC
Other									
Imp	M	1.1	1.4	3.0	3.3	0.6	0.4	0.0	0.0
	V	1.74	0.64	1.27	0.89	1.39	0.64	0.00	0.00
	n	12	5	26	21	14	10	3	3
OC	M	2.1	2.2	3.2	3.3	2.3	2.3	0.0	0.0
	V	1.38	0.90	0.66	0.59	1.19	0.81	0.00	0.00
	n	36	39	36	32	42	37	3	3
SC	M	0.1	0.2	0.4	0.4	0.2	0.1	0.0	0.0
	V	0.12	0.13	0.24	0.24	0.13	0.07	0.0	0.00
	n	36	39	36	33	44	38	3	3
Overall evaluation	M	3.4	2.5	3.1	1.8	0.5	0.8	2.5	1.5
	V	17.90	14.76	17.58	11.52	0.33	2.17	0.75	2.75
	n	36	39	36	33	44	38	4	4

The overall success of counselling was judged on a five-point scale (*0*, same; *1*, worse; *2*, some improvement; *3*, marked improvement; *4*, complete resolution). Visual inspection of the data revealed that only one patient was judged to have become worse overall; therefore, it was possible to perform an analysis of variance on the data with the scores ranging from 0 to 4 omitting the one 'worse' score.
Imp, importance; *OC*, objective change; *SC*, subjective change; *M*, means; *V*, variance

Table 47. Final Audit of Counselling: mean scores

	London	Bombay	Ibadan	Tokyo
Money				
Importance	1.26	2.42	1.39	2.50
Objective change	0.25	2.24	0.91	2.50
Subjective change	0.25	2.89	0.96	2.40
Work				
Importance	2.04	2.89	1.51	2.05
Objective change	1.38	2.93	1.22	1.75
Subjective change	1.53	3.19	1.23	1.75
Child care				
Importance	2.08	2.63	0.98	1.65
Objective change	1.31	3.38	0.87	1.0
Subjective change	1.66	3.25	0.84	1.25
Loneliness				
Importance	2.19	2.35	0.37	2.00
Objective change	1.25	2.91	0.64	2.00
Subjective change	1.36	3.11	0.68	2.00

Table 47 (Continued)

	London	Bombay	Ibadan	Tokyo
Illness/health				
Importance	2.42	2.92	3.23	1.90
Objective change	2.55	3.51	2.65	1.40
Subjective change	2.66	3.43	2.56	1.15
Bereavement				
Importance	1.00	1.49	0.62	2.00
Objective change	0.75	1.94	1.26	2.00
Subjective change	0.92	2.90	1.38	2.00
Sexual problems				
Importance	1.69	3.33	0.41	2.00
Objective change	0.98	3.20	0.57	1.65
Subjective change	1.19	3.27	0.57	1.75
Love/sexual relationships				
Importance	2.45	2.50	0.53	1.50
Objective change	1.25	2.38	0.81	1.25
Subjective change	1.43	2.42	0.77	1.25
Others				
Importance	1.24	3.19	0.49	2.00
Objective change	2.13	3.25	2.29	2.00
Subjective change	0.15	0.41	0.12	2.00

6.4.2 Overall Evaluation of Counselling

The overall success of the counselling was judged on a 5-point scale (0, same; 1, worse; 2, some improvement; 3, marked improvement; 4, complete resolution). Visual inspection of the data revealed that only one patient was judged to have become worse (score of 1) overall; therefore, it was possible to perform an analysis of variance on the data with the scores ranging from 0 to 4, omitting the one 'worse' score.

The mean scores (Tables 46 and 47) were for Bombay 2.36, for Ibadan 0.62 and for London 2.94, the differences being very highly significant ($p < 0.001$). It is clear that the Ibadan centre stands out in its negative judgement regarding the value of counselling. It is not possible to determine the success of counselling from these data, or whether these differences represent true differences among the centres or differences in the style of rating.

7 Discussion

Examination of the initial data indicates that the process of randomization generated four treatment groups which resemble each other sufficiently closely. Assessments of the result of treatment were made with the GHQ (completed by the patient) and the PSE (completed by a researcher). Previous experience with these scales has shown that they have adequate sensitivity to the effects of treatments. This has been confirmed in this trial, in which clear differences in the effects of the various treatments have appeared.

The system of dosage of diazepam was that for the first 2 weeks all patients received the same dose of 42 mg per week. General clinical experience has shown that this should be an adequate dose, somewhat on the low side. After the first 2 weeks physicians could increase the dose if they thought this necessary. In the event, the dose remained unchanged in Tokyo; there was a very slight increase in Ibadan, which in week 6 reached 44.3 mg per week, and a greater increase in London, to 49 mg per week. In Bombay the dose of drug rose quickly, and by week 6 it was almost 70 mg per week. Differences between drug dosages were very highly significant statistically ($p < 0.001$). For the last 6 weeks the dose remained about the same, except in Bombay where it fell to 62 mg per week (Table 48).

Counselling was given weekly for 6 weeks in Bombay and London, every 2 weeks for 12 weeks in Ibadan, and in Tokyo in the form of two long sessions in the first 6 weeks.

Because of the disparity between the populations sampled at the four centres, the analysis of data from the GHQ and the PSE was carried out separately for the individual centres, as well as by a four-way analysis of variance (from which Tokyo was omitted because of its few cases). Fortunately for interpretation, the results were much the same from one centre to the next.

In the above text there have been many warnings about the interpretation of tests of 'statistical significance'. These tests are very sensitive (see Sect. 5.7), and in a trial with an adequate number of patients any treatment which does not reach statistical significance may be dismissed as ineffective, by the criteria used. Even when it does prove statistically significant, judgement is required to decide whether the effect is clinically meaningful. When many tests are carried out on the same data, the criterion of 'significance' must be narrowed. As there is no universally accepted rule for this, the tests of significance have been given here in full in order to enable clinicians to judge for themselves.

Table 48. Mean weekly dose of medication (mg)

	Bombay	Ibadan	London	Tokyo	Total
Week 1					
Mean	41.3	41.3	41.6	42.0	41.5
Variance	24.44	26.64	5.41	0.0	18.68
n	104	98	85	14	301
Week 2					
Mean	40.1	41.7	41.0	42.0	41.0
Variance	59.52	24.42	28.16	0.0	36.39
n	96	96	81	14	287
Week 4					
Mean	57.9	43.7	48.2	42.0	49.6
Variance	215.6	56.47	261.09	0.0	200.54
n	86	89	75	13	263
Week 6					
Mean	66.9	44.3	49.2	42.0	52.9
Variance	215.68	64.56	272.05	0.0	262.43
n	79	84	69	13	245
Week 12					
Mean	61.7	45.7	49.5	42.0	50.1
Variance	259.14	63.80	410.56	0.0	195.39
n	37	76	13	11	137

7.1 Indirect Evaluation of Treatments

An indirect way of evaluating the treatments is to examine the rate of drop-outs. From Table 12 it can be seen that at week 6 the most drop-outs (27%) were from the placebo with no counselling group (and this was true for the individual centres of Bombay, Ibadan and Tokyo) and the least (12.8%) from the drug with no counselling group, with the placebo with counselling group (16.2%) and the drug with counselling group (14.3%) coming in between. The differences in drop-out rates are very highly significant (χ^2, 13.25; df, 3; $p < 0.005$). However, these overall figures conceal considerable differences among the four centres. The rate is highest in Tokyo (about 30%) and lowest in London (about 5%). In view of possible cultural differences, drop-out rates (if they have any meaning) are best used for within-centre comparisons. In the individual centres the lowest rates of drop-out were in either one or the other of the two drug-treated groups, with the exception of London. Here there were no drop-outs from the group receiving counselling with placebo. The rate was highest (9.8%) in the counselled group which also received drug. Although drop-out rates can be influenced by a variety of factors, these findings seem to confirm that both diazepam and counselling are effective treatments.

To the extent that drop-outs from the placebo with no counselling group was the result of dissatisfaction with treatment, the differences between active treatments and controls would be diminished. Treatments could not be distinguished by consideration of treatment-emergent symptoms. These were about the same, both in frequency and nature, in all four treatment groups.

7.2 Evaluation of Treatments with Scales

7.2.1 Effects of Treatments to Week 6

In terms of the total score on the GHQ all treatments were associated with an improvement ($p < 0.001$), with no differences between them by the end of the 2nd week. All treatments continued to show further improvement until week 6 ($p < 0.001$), but by this time counselling showed a much greater effect than no counselling. Examination of the results in the individual centres shows that this was strictly true only for Bombay ($p < 0.0001$) and was barely so for London (0.02, $p < 0.03$), but in Ibadan and Tokyo (for its four cases) the advantage of counselling, although still present, had fallen below statistically significant levels.

Factor scores show that much of the improvement occurred in factor B (anxiety and insomnia). All treatments showed highly significant improvement by week 2, but although drug did better than placebo, the difference was not significant. The advantage of counselling was clear ($p < 0.001$). By week 6 the relative merit of diazepam had diminished further ($t = 0.46$), and all treatments had continued to show further improvement, especially counselling as opposed to no counselling ($p < 0.001$). Regarding factor C (social dysfunction) all treatment groups showed steady improvement, but by week 6 that of the counselling group was only slightly better than of the no counselling group ($p < 0.05$).

The results obtained with the total score on the PSE are similar. The analysis of variance (excluding Tokyo) did show a small advantage of diazepam over placebo ($p = 0.04$) by week 6, which did not appear with the GHQ. In the analysis by individual centres, all treatments showed improvement by week 6; but whereas in Bombay counselling was better than no counselling ($p < 0.01$), and in Ibadan diazepam was barely better than placebo ($p < 0.05$), there were no differences between treatments in London.

Syndromal scores on the PSE showed somewhat conflicting results. All treatments showed the usual highly significant improvement by week 6 in all syndromal scores. Counselling was better than no counselling on all syndromal scores except 'health, worry and tension', but on 'autonomic anxiety' there was a significant interaction between counselling treatments and centre ($p = 0.014$): improvement with counselling was better than with no counselling in Bombay, about equal in Ibadan, and not as good in London. Diazepam was better than placebo for 'appetite, sleep, retardation and libido' ($p = 0.021$) and barely better for 'self and others' ($p = 0.043$). As has already been pointed out, these findings can by no means be regarded as conclusive.

7.2.2 Effects of Treatments to Weeks 6 to 12

Although the last 6 weeks of the trial was carried out on only part of the original group of patients, the evidence which is available suggests that the group which continued medication until week 12 had similar clinical scores and demographic characteristics to the group which had stopped at the 6th week. In the period between weeks 6 and 12 scores on the GHQ for all groups continued to improve ($p < 0.001$), but an analysis of variance revealed no significant differences between treatments. This is confirmed by analyses for the separate centres. Over the total period, weeks 0–12, even though the overall improvement – regardless of treatments – was highly significant, the additional advantage of counselling over no counselling was also highly significant ($p < 0.008$). In the individual centres this was true only for Bombay ($p < 0.006$), the relationship being non-significant statistically in Ibadan and London. It would seem that the advantage of counselling versus no counselling appears clearly by weeks 2 and 6 but tends to diminish thereafter.

7.3 General Improvement

All patients in this trial showed improvement, but this could not be clearly related to the specific treatments offered. There is no doubt that one of the reasons why it is difficult to demonstrate differences in the effectiveness of different treatments in psychiatry is the high rate of improvement not related to specific treatments. Furthermore, all the patients in this trial received a degree of attention and discussion of their symptoms (as part of the assessment) which was far greater than that which they would have received in everyday practice. Indeed, some patients said at the time that they felt better after the completion of the PSE. In spite of this, counselling, even of this simple and limited type, was clearly able to show benefit to the patients on most of the criteria. Of course, one must note that the assessment on the PSE was not carried out 'blind' to counselling. In Bombay, but not in Ibadan, the psychiatrists who carried out the assessments could have known which patients had been counselled, and in London it was the counsellor herself who carried them out. It might be argued that the assessments could therefore be biased in favour of counselling. Against this it can be pointed out that the results were equally clear on the GHQ scores. Although the patients knew what sort of treatment they had received, they could not know how other patients scored themselves on the questionnaire and therefore would not know how to shift the scoring of their own responses.

Drug treatment did not produce such clearly positive results. It showed some slight advantage over placebo on only some of the criteria. This cannot be ascribed to lack of sensitivity of the scales used in this trial. The simplest explanation is that it was not effective for the particular type of patient involved in this trial. Most patients complained of ill-defined symptoms, often somatic in presentation, and did not have anxiety as a dominant symptom. In contrast, most trials of anxiolytics are carried out on patients with more obviously psychological symptoms and usually with clearly diagnosable anxiety disorders. Another possible explanation is that the dosage was too low. The physicians could have increased the dose (and did so in Bombay for some of the patients), but it would appear that (in the other centres) the non-specific improvement was sufficient to make this unnecessary.

The unusual feature of this study which makes it perhaps unique among treatment trials is its combination of factors. First, it was carried out on the type of patients who are treated by general practitioners rather than by psychiatrists; second, drug treatment was crossed with psychotherapy; and, third and most important, it was a multicentre trial in which there were marked ethnocultural differences among participating centres. Counselling was offered as a first line of treatment to Africans, Asians and Europeans, literate and illiterate.

In addition, an attempt was made to examine the different procedures used in counselling and the different themes involved. Special scales were devised for this purpose, and these were able to show resemblances and differences among centres. Despite the great differences in cultural settings among the centres, there was great similarity in the methods of counselling and, surprisingly, in the themes which were discussed.

Other points worth noting are that raters were of the same cultural background as the patients; diagnoses were relatively independent of social and cultural values (although when a diagnosis was demanded, it was usually of some variety of anxiety state); and to minimize drop-outs home visits were made to carry out assessments if the patients did not come to the clinic.

7.4 Effects of the Study on Participating Centres

All those involved agreed that taking part in the study had a stimulating effect on their centres. Interest in research and transcultural problems received great encouragement, with valuable effects on clinical practice in general. In particular, the study was a great stimulus to teamwork.

7.5 Methodological Limitations

A number of limitations resulted in this study from certain features in its design and from practical problems involved in its implementation. These include the following:

1. In view of the low dosage of drug in this trial, it would have been experimentally more fruitful to have given a range of doses (low, medium, high) and to have allocated these randomly to the patients.
2. Although attempts were made for PSE assessments to be made blind to counselling (except in London), it could be argued that it would be impossible to interview a patient adequately without the rater becoming aware of the treatment received.

3. Counselling was not uniform with regard to length of sessions and the intervals between them.
4. Great difficulty was experienced in Japan with counselling. As a result the number of cases given this treatment was inadequate.
5. It was not practicable to determine the cost-effectiveness of treatment.

7.6 Further Work

The experience in this study can be used to provide the following practical suggestions for the design of future research in this area:

1. Insofar as the poor results of treatment with drug in this study could be ascribed to low dosage, a trial such as this should use higher levels of dosage.
2. It would be desirable to develop blind techniques of interviewing which are satisfactory, informative and do not reveal the nature of the treatment received. At the moment the only guarantee for blindness is a set of questions which limit the patient to replies of 'yes' or 'no'.
3. As the trial has provided good evidence that simple counselling, limited to a total of 3 h, is an effective treatment, it would be worth testing the efficacy of different systems for organizing counselling, e.g. regarding variations in the length of interviews and in their spacing.
4. Comparison of different styles of counselling, perhaps using more than one counsellor, would be worth investigating.
5. A similar trial should be carried out on patients diagnosed as suffering from anxiety states and usually treated by psychotherapists.
6. The problem of cost-effectiveness of treatment still remains to be solved.

8 Conclusions

Narratives describing findings of this study are given immediately after each section reporting results. The following four overall conclusions summarize these findings and give an assessment of feasibility of cross-cultural studies of therapeutic efficacy in common psychiatric disorders often encountered in primary health care.

(i) *Feasibility*. Although it is not mentioned as an aim of the enquiry, the practicability of such a trial was initially in question. Its successful completion has resolved all doubts concerning the difficulties of organization, the possibility of cross-cultural evaluations of drugs and counselling and, finally, the possibility of developing adequate methods for measuring the counselling process and its contents.

(ii) Drug Effects. Most of the patients admitted to this trial complained of ill-defined symptoms, often somatic in presentation, and did not have anxiety as a dominant symptom. The therapeutic effectiveness of diazepam in this type of patient is low, and less still than counselling. What effect there is lasts for not less than 6 weeks and possibly for 12, i.e. it is not short-lived. The effects appear to be much the same for different populations. Unwanted effects are not greater than those found with placebo treatment.

(iii) Counselling. Counselling is better than no counselling, and it is an effective treatment even if limited to 3 hours of counselling only.

(iv) Drug-Counselling Interaction. No significant interaction was seen between drug treatment and counselling. Thus, counselling was not significantly affected whether the patient received drug or not, and the efficacy of drug treatment was not significantly affected whether the patient received counselling or not.

References

Asberg M, Cronholm B, Sjökvist F, Tuck D (1970) Correlation of subjective side effects with plasma concentrations of nortriptyline. Br Med J [Clin Res] 4:18–21

Ban TA, Lehman HE, Galvan L, Pecknold JC, Climan M (1974) A transcultural study with clomacran: comparison of two assessment methods. Curr Therap Res Clin Exp 16(9): 971–989

Benfari RC (1969) Relationship between early dependence training and patient – therapist dyad. Psychol Rep 25:552–554

Betts TA, Clayton AB, Mackay GM (1972) Effects of four commonly used tranquilizers on low speed performance tests. Br Med J [Clin Res] 4:580–584

Bluestone H, Vela RM (1982) Transcultural aspects in the psychotherapy of the Puerto Rican poor in New York City. J Am Acad Psychoanal 10(2):269–283

Booij J (1975) Transcultural aspects of neuropsychopharmacology from the biological point of view – are they significant? In: Itil TM (ed) Transcultural neuropsychopharmacology. Bozak, Istanbul, pp 15–27

British Medical Journal (1975) Tranquilizers causing aggression. 113–114

Brown GW, Harris T (1978) The social origins of depression. A study of psychiatric disorder in women. Tavistock, London

Brown GW, Harris T, Peto J (1973a) Life events and psychiatric disorders. II: The nature of the causal link. Psychol Med 3:159–176

Brown GW, Sklair F, Harris T, Birley J (1973b) Life events and psychiatric disorders. I: Some methodological issues. Psychol Med 3:74–87

Busnello ED (1979) Psychosocial aspects of mental health care in developing countries – the role of the benzodiazepines. In: Priest RG, Vianna Filho V, Amrein R, Skreta M (eds) Benzodiazepines today and tomorrow. MTP, Lancaster, pp 203–208

Catalan J, Gath D, Edmonds G, Ennis J (1984a) The effects of non-prescribing of anxiolytics in general practice. I Controlled evaluation of psychiatric and social outcome. Br J Psychiatry 144:593–602

Catalan J, Gath D, Bond A, Martin P (1984b) The effects of non-prescribing of anxiolytics in general practice. II Factors associated with outcome. Br J Psychiatry 144:603–610

Cooper JE (1970) Use of a procedure for standardizing psychiatric diagnosis. In: Hare EH, Wing JK (eds) Psychiatric epidemiology. Oxford University Press, London

Cosmides CJ (1970) Pharmacology – toxicology. Science 168:1013–1014

Crane GE (1966) A study of psychiatric patients in Italy and USA by means of common measuring instruments. In: Brill H et al. (eds) Neuropsychopharmacology, proceedings of the fifth international congress of the Collegium Internationale Neuropsychopharmacologicum, Washington DC, 28–31 March 1966, pp 62–71

Dasberg H, van Praag HM (1974) The therapeutic effect of short-term oral diazepam treatment on acute clinical anxiety in a crisis centre. Acta Psychiatr Scand 50:326–340

Davies B, Mowbray R, Chiu E (1975) Controlled trials of doxepin (Sineguan) in Melbourne and Hong-Kong. In: Itil TM (ed) Transcultural neuropsychopharmacology. Bozak, Istanbul, pp 203–207

Day R (1981) Life events and schizophrenia – the "triggering hypothesis". Acta Psychiatr Scand 64:97–122

Denber HCB (1960) Some observations of cultural factors and their possible influence on psychiatric treatment and research. Acta Neuropsychiatr 2:212–217

Denber HCB, Bente D, Rajotte P (1962) Comparative analysis of the action of butylperazine at Manhattan State Hospital and the University Psychiatric Clinic at Erlangen. Am J Psychiatry 7:203–206

Escobar JI, Tuason VB (1980) Antidepressant agents, a cross-cultural study. Psychopharmacol Bull 16 (3):49–52
Forrest FM, Forrest IS, Serra MT (1970) Modification of chlorpromazine metabolism by some other drugs frequently administered to psychiatric patients. Biol Psychiatry 2:53–58
Forrest IS, Bookes LG, Forrest FM (1975) Some effects of induction of hepatic drug metabolizing enzymes on in vivo chlorpromazine metabolism. In: Itil TM (ed) Transcultural neuropsychopharmacology. Bozak, Istanbul, pp 55–59
Ghoneim MM, Kortilla K, Chiang CK, Jacobs L, Schoenwald RD, Mewaldt SP, Kayoba KO (1981) Diazepam effects and kinetics in Caucasians and Orientals. Clin Pharmacol Ther 29:749–756
Goldberg DP (1972) The detection of psychiatric illness by questionnaire. Oxford University Press, London
Goldberg DP, Blackwell B (1970) Psychiatric illness in a suburban general practice. A detailed study using a new method of case identification. Br Med J [Clin Res] ii:439–443
Goldberg DP, Hiller VF (1979) A scaled version of the General Health Questionnaire. Psychol Med 9:139–145
Goldberg DP, Huxley P (1980) Mental illness in the community. Tavistock, London
Goldberg DP, Kay C, Thompson L (1976) Psychiatric morbidity in general practice and the community. Psychol Med 6:565–569
Hall RCW, Joffe JR (1972) Aberrant response to diazepam. A new syndrome. Am J Psychiatry 129:738–742
Hamilton M (1975) Transcultural aspects of neuropsychopharmacology from the methodological point of view. In: Itil TM (ed) Transcultural neuropsychopharmacology. Bozak, Istanbul, pp 185–186
Harding TW, Chrusciel TL (1975) The use of psychotropic drugs in developing countries. Bull WHO 52:357–367
Hawton K, Blackstock E (1976) General practice aspects of self-poisoning and self-injury. Psychol Med 6:571–575
Hayes SL, Pablo G, Radomski T, Palmer RF (1977) Ethanol and oral diazepam abortion. N Eng J Med 296:186–189
Itil TM (1975) Transcultural psychopharmacology from the EEG point of view. In: Itil TM (ed) Transcultural neuropsychopharmacology. Bozak, Istanbul, pp 39–54
Itil TM, Reisberg B (1977) Transcultural aspects of psychopharmacology. Curr Psychiatr Ther 17:325–332
Joyce CRB (1975) Methodological aspects of a multicentre (international) trial of a new antidepressive Ciba 34, 276 – Ba. In: Itil TM (ed) Transcultural neuropsychopharmacology. Bozak, Istanbul, pp 209–215
Joyce CRB (1980) Cultural variation in the responses to pharmacotherapy and the "non-specific" factors which may affect this. Transcultural Psychiatr Res 17:129–148
Kedward H (1969) The outcome of neurotic illness in the community. Soc Psychiatry 4: 1–4
Kendell RE, Everitt B, Cooper JE, Sartorius N, David ME (1968) Reliability of the present state examination. Soc Psychiatry 3:123
Kleinman A (1981) Culture and patient care: psychiatry among the Chinese. Drug Ther ii (11):134–135, 138–140
Kortilla K, Mattila MJ, Linnoila M (1976) Prolonged recovery after diazepam sedation – the influence of food, charcoal ingestion and injection rate on the effects of intravenous diazepam. Br J Anaesth 48:333–340
Krause MS, Howard KI (1983) Design and analysis issues in the cross-cultural evaluation of psychotherapies. Cult Med Psychiatry 7(3):301–311
Ladewig D (1983) Abuse of benzodiazepines in western European society – incidence and prevalence, motives and drug acquisition. Pharmacopsychiatry 16:103–106
Ladewig D (1984) Dependence liability of the benzodiazepines. Drug Alcohol Depend 13:139–149
Lin KM, Poland RE, Lesser IM (1986) Ethnicity and psychopharmacology. Cult Med Psychiatry 10:151–165
Marcos LR, Cancro R (1982) Pharmacotherapy of Hispanic depressed patients: clinical observations. Am J Psychother 36(4):505–512

Murphy HBM (1969) Ethnic variation in drug response. Transcultural Psychiatr Res 6:5–23
Murphy HBM (1975) The meaning of culture for psychopharmacological research. In: Itil TM (ed) Transcultural neuropsychopharmacology. Bozak, Istanbul, pp 7–13
Newson-Smith JGB, Hirsch SR (1979) Psychiatric symptoms in self-poisoning patients. Psychol Med 9:493–500
Okuma T (1981) Differential sensitivity to the effects of psychotropic drugs: psychotics versus normals; Asian versus Western populations. Jpn J Psychiatry Neurol 35(1):79–87
Olatawura MO (1976) An uncontrolled clinical trial with clomipramine (Anafranil) in the treatment of depressed Nigerian patients. Afr J Psychiatry 2:315–318
Olatawura MO (1977) Effectiveness of psychotropic drugs in patients in a state of malnutrition or exposed to extreme climatic conditions. Psychopharmacol Bull 13(1):8–13
Petursson H, Lader MH (1981) Withdrawal from long-term benzodiazepine treatment. Br Med J [Clin Res] 283:643–645
Prescott LF (1983) Safety of the benzodiazepines. In: Costa E (ed) Benzodiazepines from molecular biology to clinical practice. Raven, New York, pp 253–265
Priest RG (1980) The benzodiazepines: a clinical review. In: Priest RG, Filho UV, Amrein R, Skreta M (eds) Benzodiazepines today and tomorrow. MTP Lancaster, pp 77–83
Raskin A, Crook I (1975) Antidepressants in black and white in-patients. Differential response to a controlled trial of chlorpromazine and imipramine. Arch Gen Psychiatry 32:643
Rickels K (1968) Non-specific factors in drug therapy. Thomas, Illinois
Rickels K, Downing RW (1970) Drug and placebo treated neurotic out-patients. Arch Gen Psychiatry 16:369–372
Salzman C, Kochansky GE, Shadder RI, Porrino LJ, Harmatz JS, Swift CP (1974) Chlordiazepoxide – induced hostility in a small group setting. Arch Gen Psychiatry 31:401–405
Sartorius N (1973) Culture and epidemiology of depression. Psychiatria Neurol Neurchir 75:479–487
Sartorius N (1978) The new mental health programme of WHO. Interdisciplinary Sci Rev 3:202–206
Sartorius N (1983) Collaborative studies. Exp Clin Psychiatry 7:487–504
Sartorius N, Jablensky A, Shapiro R (1977) Two-year follow-up of the patients included in the WHO International Pilot Study on Schizophrenia. Psychol Med 7, 529–541
Schlesinger R (1981) Cross-cultural psychiatry: the applicability of Western Anglo psychiatry to Asian – Americans of Chinese and Japanese ethnicity. J Psychosoc Nurs Ment Health Serv 19(9):26–30
Seppala T, Kortilla K, Hakkinen S, Linnoila M (1976) Residual effects and skills related to driving after a single oral administration of diazepam, medazepam or lorazepam. Br J Clin Pharmacol 3: 831–841
Shepherd M, Cooper B, Brown AC, Kalton G (1981) Psychiatric illness in general practice, 2nd ed. Oxford University Press, London
Simeon J (1975) Evaluation of therapeutic responses in different cultures: problems of methodology. In: Itil TM (ed) Transcultural neuropsychopharmacology. Bozak, Istanbul, pp 187–191
Takahashi R, Nakane Y, Akiyama A (1979) Lithium treatment in affective disorders from viewpoint of transcultural psychopharmacology: therapeutic plasma level. Jpn J Psychiatry Neurol 33(4):501–509
Ulett GA, Ulett PC (1975) A standardized system of psychiatry in transcultural studies. In: Itil TM (ed) Transcultural neuropsychopharmacology. Bozak, Istanbul, pp 197–202
Vartanian FE (1979a) World Health Organization activity in psychopharmacotherapy. In: Progress Neuropsychopharmacology. vol 3. Pergamon, Oxford, pp 5–9
Vartanian FE (1979b) Psychopharmacology as a subject for international collaboration. In: Cazzullo CL, Invernizzi G (eds) Prevention in psychiatry. Milano, pp 89–99
Ward J (1985) Vital uses of diazepam in third world countries. In: Smith DE, Wesson DR (eds) the benzodiazepines: current standards for medical practice. MTP Lancaster, pp 167–175
Wheatley D (1975) Transcultural problems in a domiciliary setting. In: Itil TM (ed) Transcultural neuropsychopharmacology. Bozak, Istanbul, pp 155–163
Williams P, Murray J, Clare A (1982) A longitudinal study of psychotropic drug prescription. Psychol Med 12:201–206

Wing JK, Birley JLT, Cooper JE, Graham P, Isaacs AD (1967) Reliability of a procedure for measuring and classifying "present psychiatric state". Br J Psychiatry 113:499

Wing JK et al. (1974) Measurement and classification of psychiatric symptoms. Cambridge University Press, London

Wing JK, Nixon JM, Mann SA, Leff JP (1977) Reliability of the PSE (ninth edition) used in a population study. Psychol Med 7:505–516

Winokur A, Rickel K, Greenblatt DJ, Snyder P, Schatz NJ (1980) Withdrawal reaction from long term low dosage administration of diazepam. Arch Gen Psychiatr 37:101–105

Wood D, Sherrets SD (1982/83) Race as a factor in the perceived importance of the use of psychotropic medication. J Psychiatr Res 17(3):297–301

World Health Organization (1973) The international pilot study of schizophrenia, vol 1. WHO, Geneva

World Health Organization (1976) Drug treatment for neuropsychiatric disorders in developing countries: report on a consultation. OMH/76.2. WHO, Geneva

World Health Organization (1979) Schizophrenia, an international follow-up study. Wiley, New York

World Health Organization (1980) Psychopharmacology – an area of research to improve mental health care. WHO Chron 34:465–469

World Health Organization (1981) Social dimension of mental health. WHO, Geneva

World Health Organization (1982) WHO seventh general programme of work. WHO, Geneva

World Health Organization (1986) Dose effects of antidepressant medication in different populations. J Affective Disord Suppl 2:S1–S67

Yamashita I, Asano Y (1979) Tricyclic antidepressants therapeutic plasma level. Psychopharmacol Bull 15(4):40–41

Appendix A: Description of Research Centres and Study Areas

A.1 Description of Research Centre and Study Area of Bombay

A.1.1 Description of Centre/Catchment Area

A.1.1.1 Geographical Characteristics of Bombay City

Bombay, the capital city of Maharasthra State and the commercial centre of India is a cosmopolitan, metropolitan island with a maximum width of 8 km and connected to the mainland at its broad northern end. It has a total area of 433.71 km^2 and an estimated population of 8 243 000. The average density of the population is 18 833/km^2 although in the south the density is 47 810/km^2, one of the highest in the world. Its population increases every day (in addition to birth) by the arrival of some 1500 persons from other parts of the country seeking jobs and better living. Although families of the younger generation move from the city out to the suburbs, the population continues to increase in all parts of Bombay in the form of the new slums that sprout at times.

A.1.1.2 Economy and Employment

Textiles constitute the main industry located in the island part of the city. Chemical, pharmaceutical, engineering, metal, oil and fertilizer industries are other important industries that are located in the suburbs and extended suburbs. Nearly 60% of all industry in Maharasthra State is located in Bombay. To prevent additional influx into the city, new industries are encouraged to locate in the twin city, New Bombay, which is located on the coastal area of the mainland. Manufacturing employs 55% of the population; nearly 45% is engaged in the service sector and a negligible number of people are occupied in agriculture.

A.1.1.3 Family Structure and Housing

Shortage of housing has led to appalling living conditions. Some 80% of inhabitants live in one-room tenements without basic facilities, and 50% live with three to five persons per room, with less than 40 ft^2 (3.7 m^2) of living space for each individual. Only 28% of the people have independent water taps – with an erratic water supply – while the rest depend on community taps. This overcrowding leads to many unhealthy personal and social consequences.

Noise and air pollution is very high due to traffic congestion and the fertilizer industry located in Bombay. Transport is difficult due to the geographical linearity of the city, and people spend an average of 4 h travelling to and from their workplaces, located mostly in the south of the city.

The social structure of Bombay does not follow the same geographical pattern as that in major Western cities. Rather than in terms of economic status or social class, districts of the city are organized more on the basis of caste, religion and language, cutting across the social, economic, educational and occupational divisions.

A.1.1.4 Population and Education

The total population of Bombay in 1981 stood at 8243000. Of the city's inhabitants 56% are men and 44% women.

The literacy rate in greater Bombay, at 68.2%, compares very favourably to the rate for India as a whole, which is estimated at 36.1%. While men have a higher literacy rate in Bombay than do women, the differences between the sexes in this regard are not as great as in the rest of the country. Male literacy in greater Bombay is estimated at 74.0% and female literacy at 60.6%, while the corresponding figures for all of India are 46.6% and 24.7%.

A.1.2 Description of the Facility at the Centre

A.1.2.1 Medical and Psychiatric Services

The medical services in the area include 25 general hospitals (20 supported by municipality, three by the state government and two by the central government), two general hospitals for the railways, four state insurance hospitals (mostly for labourers), 13 maternity hospitals, and two general hospitals for children. There are some ten private general hospitals and one general hospital for cancer. Health care is also provided by 154 municipal dispensaries, eight mobile dispensaries and 33 dental clinics.

Three municipal general hospitals and one government general hospital maintain the four medical colleges in Bombay; these admit about 600 new students for undergraduate and some 400–500 for post-graduate medical studies each year. These medical colleges are connected with the University of Bombay, one of the oldest in the country.

Medical services in Bombay are of three types. (a) The municipal and government hospitals and the dispensaries give medical advice and treatment to everyone who seeks help, almost free of, or for only a nominal, charge. Generally, people of lower socioeconomic status seek help here. About 10%–20% of patients come from outside Bombay. (b) For employees, the state insurance system offers medical help through its general hospitals, special dispensaries and diagnostic centres. It also looks after individual employees by means of a yearly contract with general medical practitioners, each of whom tends to some 1000–1500 families. (c) Private medical practices are prevalent and well-organized.

A rough estimate of the number of doctors in Bombay working in the various categories is as follows:

General practitioners	13000	Gynaecologists and obstetricians	400
Surgeons	300		
Physicians	350	Paediatricians	225

Psychiatrists	70	Anaesthesiologists	200
Dermatologists	60	Dental surgeons	400
Otorhinolaryngologists	110	Ophthalmologists	100
Neurologists and neurosurgeons	25	Orthopaedic surgeons	80
Pathologists	300		
Plastic surgeons	20		

There are about 60 psychiatrists in private practice in Bombay. Of these, 20 serve as honorary professors of psychiatry in the four teaching hospitals attached to the University of Bombay. General hospital psychiatry is the dominant form of psychiatric help that has evolved in the city of Bombay. A large majority of patients seek help from the general hospital psychiatric departments. There are in all 210 in-patient beds in these hospitals.

In addition, a mental hospital maintained by the state government with about 1000 beds is located in a major town, Thane, outside greater Bombay. This offers a long-term facility to chronic psychotics of the city of Bombay and the Thane district.

A.1.2.2 Department of Psychiatry, King Edward VII Memorial Hospital and Seth G.S. Medical College affiliated to University of Bombay

This in-patient service provides 60 beds and has 1000–1100 admissions per year. Out-patient services for adults include some 6600 out-patients and 33 700 consultations annually and those for children some 800 out-patients and 4900 consultations. The out-patient service is open every day, with three honorary professors giving consultations. There is a 24-h casualty walk-in service. The staff of the Department of Psychiatry comprises the following: one emeritus professor of psychiatry, two honorary professors of psychiatry, one honorary associate professor, three honorary assistant professors, two lecturers in psychiatry, five senior residents in psychiatry (registrars), four junior residents (house physicians), two clinical psychologists, two psychiatric social workers, six occupational therapists, and ten nurses.

The general policy in the Department for the past 25 years has been one of short-term hospitalization of acute or severe psychotics, acute or severe depressives or suicidal patients, acute hysterical conversion reactions, etc. In-patient stay per patient is generally 7–14 days. Those with diagnostic problems or psychosomatic disorders are admitted for comprehensive evaluation. The types of treatment given by the Department are psychopharmacotherapy, electroconvulsive therapy, brief psychotherapy of a problem-oriented and supportive type, behaviour therapy, group educational therapy, family case work, educative counselling, child guidance therapy, and occupational therapy.

Referrals from other branches of medicine and consultation-liaison psychiatry form part of the routine activity of the Department. Nearly one-third of patients are referred by other medical departments. Teaching of undergraduate medical students, training of post-graduate students in psychiatry, teaching of nurses, physiotherapists, occupational therapists and psychiatric social workers also belong to the routine activities of the Department.

The research conducted here is largely clinical and consists of psychosocial and phenomenological study of major and minor psychiatric conditions, including psychosomatic disorders such as diabetes mellitus and mucous colitis. Treatment research is a regular feature and consists of evaluation of psychopharmacotherapy, electroconvulsive therapy, psychotherapy, behaviour therapy, etc. in various psychiatric conditions. Schizophrenias, depressions, alcoholism and neuroses are the four conditions which receive priority in research. Newer areas of research include the detection and management of psychiatric problems in patients attending medical, dermatological, gynaecological and obstetric, and otorhinolaryngological services, as well as a study of dying and death-related problems.

A.1.3 Description of Recruitment and Treatment Procedures

For selection as subjects in the present study, all patients attending the psychiatric out-patient service of our Department and diagnosed as suffering from minor psychoneurotic problems were seen by a senior resident, and each was given the Need-for-Treatment Scale. Only those patients needing minor anxiolytics and/or counselling and not needing hospitalization or antidepressants were interviewed. Those living far away from the Department, those who could not come for regular evaluations are required, those already on psychotropic drugs, or those with alcohol or drug problems were excluded. The GHQ was administered to the remaining patients by the researcher, and those scoring 12 or more were included in the study.

A.2 Description of Research Centre and Study Area of Ibadan

A.2.1 Description of Centre/Catchment Area

A.2.1.1 Geographical Characteristics of Ibadan City

Ibadan is the administrative centre of Oyo State, one of the 19 states which make up the Federal Republic of Nigeria. It lies some 140 km northeast of the capital city of Lagos, in the southwestern part of the country. Ibadan appears to grow every day and now covers an area of some 150 km^2. Although no reliable census data are available, a 2.5% growth rate projection on the 1963 census put the 1979 population of Ibadan at 931 348. By now, this figure will have passed the one-million mark.

Ibadan has both urban and 'suburban' characteristics. The more affluent sector of the city, occupied by 'non-natives', is urban while the suburban area is in many respects rural and is occupied largely by the true Ibadans. The urban part lies in the west and the suburban part in the east of the city. The latter is characterized by over-crowding, particularly during festivals, e.g. Muslim festivals, when Ibadans return to the city from their farms, which can be as far as 25 km away.

A.2.1.2 Economy and Employment

Because Ibadan has been an important administrative centre since colonial days, it has attracted mainly white-collar workers, employed in government offices, commercial firms, and secondary and higher institutions of learning. The past 15 years or so, however, have witnessed the growth of the industrial sector. Industries located in Ibadan include beer and soft-drinks producers, plastic wares and utensils factories, and steel works. The latter manufactures mainly household furniture. Most of the jobs here are taken by non-natives, while natives engage in farming, driving motor-vehicles, petty trading and low-paid jobs in factories and offices. A very rough estimate shows that about 75% of the labour force is employed in the service sector, some 14% in industry and trading and about 1% in farming. There is some 10% unemployment.

A.2.1.3 Family Structure and Housing

The usual family structure is the traditional extended family system. Although there is a high infant mortality rate, particularly in the suburban area, the average number of children per woman is four. The marriage pattern is polygynous. Traditional households or family compounds are very common in the native sector. The urban sector is characterized by single-room lodgings for single clerks and apartments of up to three bedrooms for more senior married office workers. There is much over-crowding in the native areas, and dwellings in the urban sector may also have as many as two to three persons per room.

A.2.1.4 Population and Education

The catchment area of the University College Hospital coincides roughly with the city of Ibadan. Being a teaching/specialist hospital, some 2% of patients in the General Out-patient Department come from outside Ibadan.

According to the estimated 1979 census, out of a total population of 931 348, males account for 57% of the population. The population in Ibadan by age and sex (1979) is as follows:

Age group	Men	Women	Totals
0–19	181 751	159 932	341 683
20–44	313 986	211 900	525 886
45–54	22 155	16 838	37 993
55+	141 026	11 760	25 786

Ibadan is a university city, the seat of the oldest university and teaching hospital in the country. There are some twenty secondary schools, two teacher-training colleges and a polytechnic. Despite these educational institutions, there is a high level of illiteracy (20%), especially in the native, suburban part of the city. There are no minority groups as such in Ibadan.

A.2.2 Description of Facilities at the Centre

A.2.2.1 Medical and Psychiatric Services

Ibadan has a 500-bed university teaching hospital supported by the federal government, two state general hospitals, some eight maternity units and a school of hygiene. There is also an armed forces hospital in the city. The city is covered with numerous private clinics, operated mostly on a part-time basis by doctors just starting their careers or with full-time positions in government and industry. There are some 200 doctors working in the city, but most of these are located in the teaching hospital. A rough estimate of the numbers of the different categories of doctors working in Ibadan is:

General practitioners (full time)	20	Ophthalmologists	5
Surgeons	28	Neurologists and neurosurgeons	5
Gynaecologists	22	Dermatologists	1
Physicians	25	Otorhinolaryngologists	7
Paediatricians	15	Psychiatrists	5

The rest of the large number of about 200 doctors is made up of specialists such as those in pathology, public health and anaesthesia and by general duty doctors and trainees of various grades. The government (federal and state) services and private clinics provide about 3000 beds for the population of Ibadan.

A.2.2.2 Department of Psychiatry, University College Hospital Ibadan

There are only nine beds allocated to the Department of Psychiatry in the 500-bed University Teaching Hospital. The Department is thus well-known for its out-patient and domiciliary forms of psychiatric management. For its in-patient services, the Aro Village Therapeutic Community and the Aro Neuro-Psychiatric Hospital, both at Abeokuta, meet this deficiency. There is also active collaboration between the Department and the state psychiatric unit in the city some 10 km away.

The staff of the Department of Psychiatry includes four consultant psychiatrists, four senior house officer/registrar grades, two senior registrars, two social workers, and five trained psychiatric nurses.

The type of treatment offered includes psychopharmacotherapy, electroconvulsive therapy, short-term problem-focused psychotherapy, occupational therapy and day-care support.

There is a Behavioural Sciences Research Unit attached to the Department. This unit has a staff of eight very experienced research nursing officers. Research activities include studies of outcome of severe mental disorders, drug abuse, student health, child and adolescent adjustment problems, depression and psychotropic drugs in African populations.

A.2.3 Description of Recruitment and Treatment Procedures

Patients for the present study were recruited from the General Out-patient Department of the University Teaching Hospital. Inclusion criteria were discussed with the head of the Department and with the research team. Those judged by the general practitioners as suitable were referred to the team of research nursing officers who were usually present every morning. The patients who were thought suitable by the research nursing officers were then brought to the Department a short distance away. The final decision to include any patient in the study was made by the research psychiatrist. The patients were randomly assigned to the treatment modalities according to a previous research plan. Two nursing officers were specially trained to administer counselling as required by the research protocol in a selected room. Once admitted to the study, subjects were seen exclusively by the departmental research team until the end of the study.

A.3 Description of Research Centre and Study Area of London

A.3.1 Description of Centre/Catchment Area

The study was carried out in the surgeries (offices) of the three general practice groups, two in the borough of Hammersmith and Fulham and one in the borough of Kingston. The borough of Hammersmith is a mixed area in terms of social class, with a preponderance of skilled labour but also containing sizeable populations of manual labour and the middle class. The two surgeries are placed in parts of the borough where they received a mixed population. The third practice, in Barnes, serves a mainly middle-class population including professionals, businessmen, actors, artists, etc. All three are group practices with three to five general practitioners each. There are receptionists and a nurse on the premises, and the practice is assisted by a health visitor who combines the functions of a nurse and a social worker and by district community nurses. At times counsellors have assisted the practitioners.

General practitioners are private contractors to the National Health Service, which pays the practitioners on a per-capita basis for each patient registered on their lists, whether the patient is treated during the year or not. There are no payments for specific items of service, except for certain items such as vaccinations, health smears and pap smears, and the doctor does not receive more if he sees a patient several times rather than only once. Patients come normally by appointment, but there are times in the day when they can come on a 'first come, first served' basis. How the practice is organized in this respect is a matter for each practice.

While the general practitioners are aware of psychiatric issues, the majority do not have psychiatry as a special interest, and their training in this area of medical practice may be minimal.

A.3.2 Description of Facilities at the Centre

The research was carried out by the academic Department of Psychiatry of Charing Cross Hospital Medical School. This department has five full-time academic staff including a professor, two readers and two lecturers (at the time of the study), and there are five consultant psychiatrists, including one child psychiatrist, and six psychiatric trainees. There are up to a dozen attached research workers and external students, some of whom are on research grants from other research bodies. The Department of Psychiatry has 40 beds and sees approximately 12000 out-patient visits per year, of which 2500 are new referrals. They carry out about 1000 consultations per year on the general medical and surgical wards. The orientation of the Department is mainly biological, i.e. using medication, but electroconvulsive therapy and also some forms of psychotherapy and behaviour therapy are practized by the psychologists. There is a day hospital which is devoted to the improvement of patients' personal functioning, and the hospital is backed up by a mental hospital which takes a few cases each year of patients who have not responded to treatment. The facilities of this hospital are all part of the National Health Service, and patients pay neither at the general practice nor, if they have a referral, to the Department of Psychiatry. Research in the Department is focused on schizophrenia, liaison psychiatry and psychosomatic medicine and psychopharmacology. Social psychiatry and administrative issues are other areas of interest as is research into psychotherapy, benzodiazepines and the psychophysiology of hypnosis.

Patients are admitted to the psychiatric unit by their general practitioner, or they are referred by accident and emergency departments or other out-patient departments. A few are admitted following a domiciliary visit, requested by the general practitioner or the social services and carried out by senior medical staff.

A.3.3 Description of Recruitment and Treatment Procedures

Recruitment for the study occurred in one of two ways. Either the general practitioner identified the patient whom he thought had a possible emotional component to his complaint and might respond to counselling or benzodiazepines, or the patient was identified by routine screening using the GHQ; this is a self-administered questionnaire that patients filled out while waiting in the waiting room at the request of the research worker. Patients with high scores, suggesting possible emotional problems, were brought to the general practitioner's attention and where appropriate were referred for inclusion in the study.

A.4 Description of Research Centre and Study Area of Tokyo

A.4.1 Description of Centre/Catchment Area

A.4.1.1 Geographical Characteristics of Ichikawa City

The Tokyo centre is located in Ichikawa City, adjacent to Tokyo Metropolitan City and with 386823 inhabitants (196722 men and 190101 women) in 1983. It has a total area of 56.31 km^2, and the average density of the population is 6870/km^2. The population increased in 1983 by 1.8%. The city is a traditional, old town dating from the fifteenth century, and its population consists mainly of white-collar employees who commute into Tokyo.

A.4.1.2 Economy and Employment

The city is mainly a residential area, i.e. a 'bedroom' suburb of Tokyo City. The number of its inhabitants working inside the city itself is 91 109. Of these, 32.8% are employed in wholesale and retail trades, 26.9% in manufacturing industry and 16.9% in the service sector.

A.4.1.3 Family Structure and Housing

In 1983 the birth and mortality rates were 1.56% and 0.4%, whilst marriage and divorce rates were 0.82% and 18.8%, respectively. The percentage of foreign residents in the city was only 0.2%, 70% of whom were Koreans. For its 386 823 inhabitants there were 138 166 households, i.e. an average of 2.8 persons per household. As in any other urban area in Japan, the number of extended families is decreasing while that of nuclear families is increasing. Although the rate of population increase fell from 6.1% in 1963 to 1.8% in 1983, the population density has increased from 3381/km^2 in 1963 to 6870/km^2 in 1983.

A.4.1.4 Population and Education

The percentage of the population in Ichikawa City (1980) aged 65 or over is 5.8%, which is lower than the 8.8% figure in the general population.

The population in Ichikawa City by age and sex is as follows:

Age group	Men	Women	Totals
0–19	57985	55274	113169
20–44	87368	80329	167169
45–54	19965	19220	39185
55+	19123	24225	43348

Ichikawa is a university town and has three universities and three colleges with a total of 10 304 students. There are 264 kindergartens, 978 primary schools, 15 high schools and eight other special schools.

A.4.2 Description of the Facilities at the Centre

A.4.2.1 Medical and Psychiatric Services

Ichikawa has 19 hospitals with 3182 beds. Among these, there are two mental hospitals and a Department of Psychiatry in the general hospital with a total of 1059 psychiatric beds. There are 382 doctors (among them 37 psychiatrists), 221 dentists, 522 nurses, 56 midwives and 533 pharmacists in the city.

Ichikawa Prefectural Health Centre was established in 1944 with 51 staff members. These carry out mental health counselling, consultation services for the elderly, day-care treatment for the mentally ill, home visits, consultation for alcoholics and the organizing of meetings for relatives of the mentally ill.

A.4.2.2 National Institute of Mental Health and Konodai National Hospital

The Centre is located at the National Institute of Mental Health, which is the only national research and training centre for mental health in Japan. The Institute is supported and supervised by the Ministry of Health and Welfare. The National Institute of Mental Health has seven departments, those for Child Mental Health, Adult Mental Health, Psychogeriatrics, Psychophysiological Study, Human Genetics, Socioenvironmental Research, and Mental Retardation Research. It also runs an out-patient clinic and day-care centre for both adults and children.

It cooperates with Konodai National General Hospital, located in the same premises as the Institute. This provides 800 beds, of which 400 are for psychiatric patients. In 1983 the hospital treated 224634 in-patients, among whom 105445 were psychiatric patients. However, over 50% of these patients were living in Tokyo, because transportation from the centre of Tokyo City is very convenient, taking only 20 min from Tokyo Central Station to Ichikawa Station.

A.4.2.3 Other Mental Health Resources

Ichikawa has a city child guidance clinic, city council for the prevention of delinquency, a private institution for the mentally retarded and several classes for retarded children. Among instances of delinquent behaviour stealing accounts for 70%.

A.4.3 Description of Recruitment and Treatment Procedures

Almost all the patients included in the present study were out-patients at the Konodai National Hospital or a private mental hospital. All were inhabitants of the city. Patients were seen by psychiatrists, who made the diagnosis and determined whether they were suitable for inclusion in the study. Only those scoring 11 or more on the GHQ were included in the study, this differing from the cut-off point of 12 at other centres. Once they had been informed and had given approval for participation, those assigned to the group receiving counselling were referred to clinical psychologists with 5 or more years of experience at counselling.

Appendix B: Data Collection Forms

GENERAL HEALTH QUESTIONNAIRE

Note to the Researcher

Investigator should complete the schedule after the patient has answered all questions.

In Section 2, two rating scales are required for each question: in the first scale marked "Screening", any answer in the first two columns will be rated "0". Investigator rates "1" for any of the questions with an answer in the third or fourth column.

In the second scale marked "Scoring", any answer in the first column will be rated "0". Investigator rates "1" for any of the questions with an answer in the second column, "2" for answer in the third column and "3" for answer in the fourth column.

Please enter the appropriate code in the boxes provided on the right hand margin and enter the total score below. Only patients with a total score of 12 or more in the "Screening" scale would be included in the study.

Sample:

					Screening	Scoring
– been feeling perfectly well and in good health?	Better than usual	(Same as usual)	Worse than usual	Much worse than usual	0	1
– been feeling in need of a good tonic?	Not at all	No more than usual	(Rather more than usual)	Much more than usual	1	2

Section 1 – Identification / Decision on Inclusion or Exclusion Ø M B P 2 5 0 1 01-08

Study Centre No.:

02 = Bombay
08 = Ibadan
09 = London
10 = Tokyo

☐☐ 09-10

Name of Researcher who Interviewed this Patient: ____________ ☐☐ (leave blank) 11-12

0 0 0 13-15

Patient's Registration Number in Facility: ____________

Patient's WHO Number: To be filled in later if the patient is definitely included ☐☐☐ 16-18

Date of Interview: Day Month Year ☐☐☐☐☐☐ 19-24

Total Score: Screening ☐☐ Scoring ☐☐

If patient EXCLUDED: **Please keep these forms for subsequent return to WHO in Geneva.**

If patient INCLUDED: **Please fill in patient's WHO number, add these forms after completion to the Patient Documentation and continue with the interview.**

Section 2 – Physical Data

Height: in centimeters ☐☐☐ 25-27

Body Weight: in kilograms ☐☐☐ 28-30

Pulse Rate: beats/min. ☐☐☐ 31-33

Blood Pressure: in mmHg

Sitting position: Systolic ☐☐☐ Diastolic ☐☐☐ 34-39

The Effects of Benzodiazepines and Therapeutic Counselling in Different Populations

Screening Interview / Interview No. 1

ØMBP2501

Please read this carefully:

We should like to know if you have any **medical complaints**, and how your health has been in general, **over the past few weeks**. Please answer all the questions in the following pages simply by **putting a circle** around the answer which you think most nearly applies to you. Remember that we want to know about **present and recent complaints**, not those that you had in the past.

It is important to try **to answer all** the questions.

Thank you very much for your cooperation.

Write your – Name:

– Home Address:

Do not write in this space

Sex: (circle the appropriate) Male Female — 46

How old are you? — 47-48

Status: (circle the appropriate) Single Married Widowed Separated Divorced — 49

Have you recently

						Screening	Scoring	
1.	– **been feeling perfectly well and in good health?**	Better than usual	Same as usual	Worse than usual	Much worse than usual			50
2.	– **been feeling in need of a good tonic?**	Not at all	No more than usual	Rather more than usual	Much more than usual			51
3.	– **been feeling run down and out of sorts?**	Not at all	No more than usual	Rather more than usual	Much more than usual			52
4.	– **felt that you are ill?**	Not at all	No more than usual	Rather more than usual	Much more than usual			53
5.	– **been getting any pains in your head?**	Not at all	No more than usual	Rather more than usual	Much more than usual			54
6.	– **been getting a feeling of tightness or pressure in your head?**	Not at all	No more than usual	Rather more than usual	Much more than usual			55
7.	– **been able to concentrate on whatever you're doing?**	Better than usual	Same as usual	Less than usual	Much less than usual			56
8.	– **been afraid that you were going to collapse in a public place?**	Not at all	No more than usual	Rather more than usual	Much more than usual			57
9.	– **been having hot or cold spells?**	Not at all	No more than usual	Rather more than usual	Much more than usual			58
10.	– **been perspiring (sweating) a lot?**	Not at all	No more than usual	Rather more than usual	Much more than usual			59
11.	– **found yourself waking early and**	Not	No more	Rather more	Much more			60

World Health Organization

The Effects of Benzodiazepines and Therapeutic Counselling in Different Populations

Screening Interview / Interview No. 1

ØMBP2501

						Do not write in this space Screening	Scoring	
12.	– **been getting up feeling your sleep hasn't refreshed you?**	Not at all	No more than usual	Rather more than usual	Much more than usual			61
13.	– **been feeling too tired and exhausted even to eat?**	Not at all	No more than usual	Rather more than usual	Much more than usual			62
14.	– **lost much sleep over worry?**	Not at all	No more than usual	Rather more than usual	Much more than usual			63
15.	– **been feeling mentally alert and wide awake?**	Better than usual	Same as usual	Less than usual	Much less than usual			64
16.	– **been feeling full of energy?**	Better than usual	Same as usual	Less energy than usual	Much less energetic			65
17.	– **had difficulty in getting off to sleep?**	Not at all	No more than usual	Rather more than usual	Much more than usual			66
18.	– **had difficulty in staying asleep once you are off?**	Not at all	No more than usual	Rather more than usual	Much more than usual			67
19.	– **been having frightening or unpleasant dreams?**	Not at all	No more than usual	Rather more than usual	Much more than usual			68
20.	– **been having restless, disturbed nights?**	Not at all	No more than usual	Rather more than usual	Much more than usual			69
21.	– **been managing to keep yourself busy and occupied?**	More so than usual	Same as usual	Rather less than usual	Much less than usual			70
22.	– **been taking longer over the things you do?**	Quicker than usual	Same as usual	Longer than usual	Much longer than usual			71
23.	– **tended to lose interest in your ordinary activities?**	Not at all	No more than usual	Rather more than usual	Much more than usual			72
24.	– **been losing interest in your personal appearance?**	Not at all	No more than usual	Rather more than usual	Much more than usual			73
25.	– **been taking less trouble with your clothes?**	More trouble than usual	About same as usual	Less trouble than usual	Much less trouble			74
26.	– **been getting out of the house as much as usual?**	More than usual	Same as usual	Less than usual	Much less than usual			75
27.	– **been managing as well as most people would in your shoes?**	Better than most	About the same	Rather less well	Much less well			76
28.	– **felt on the whole you were doing things well?**	Better than usual	About the same	Less well than usual	Much less well			77
29.	– **been late getting to work or getting started on your housework?**	Not at all	No later than usual	Rather later than usual	Much later than usual			78
30.	– **been satisfied with the way you've carried out your task?**	More satisfied	About same as usual	Less satisfied than usual	Much less satisfied			79
						ØMBP2502		01-08
31.	– **been able to feel warmth and affection to those near to you?**	Better than usual	About same as usual	Less well than usual	Much less well			19
32.	– **been finding it easy to get on with other people?**	Better than usual	About same as usual	Less well than usual	Much less well			20
33.	– **spent much time chatting with**	More time	About same	Less	Much less			21

Do not write in this space

						Screening	Scoring	
34.	**– kept feeling afraid to say anything to people in case you made a fool of yourself?**	Not at all	No more than usual	Rather more than usual	Much more than usual	☐	☐	22
35.	**– felt that you are playing a useful part in things?**	More so than usual	Same as usual	Less useful than usual	Much less useful	☐	☐	23
36.	**– felt capable of making decisions about things?**	More so than usual	Same as usual	Less so than usual	Much less capable	☐	☐	24
37.	**– felt you're just not able to make a start on anything?**	Not at all	No more than usual	Rather more than usual	Much more than usual	☐	☐	25
38.	**– felt yourself dreading everything that you have to do?**	Not at all	No more than usual	Rather more than usual	Much more than usual	☐	☐	26
39.	**– felt constantly under strain?**	Not at all	No more than usual	Rather more than usual	Much more than usual	☐	☐	27
40.	**– felt you couldn't overcome your difficulties?**	Not at all	No more than usual	Rather more than usual	Much more than usual	☐	☐	28
41.	**– been finding life a struggle all the time?**	Not at all	No more than usual	Rather more than usual	Much more than usual	☐	☐	29
42.	**– been able to enjoy your normal day-to-day activities?**	More so than usual	Same as usual	Less so than usual	Much less than usual	☐	☐	30
43.	**– been taking things hard?**	Not at all	No more than usual	Rather more than usual	Much more than usual	☐	☐	31
44.	**– been getting edgy and bad-tempered?**	Not at all	No more than usual	Rather more than usual	Much more than usual	☐	☐	32
45.	**– been getting scared or panicky for no good reason?**	Not at all	No more than usual	Rather more than usual	Much more than usual	☐	☐	33
46.	**– been able to face up to your problems?**	More so than usual	Same as usual	Less able than usual	Much less able	☐	☐	34
47.	**– found everything getting on top of you?**	Not at all	No more than usual	Rather more than usual	Much more than usual	☐	☐	35
48.	**– had the feeling that people were looking at you?**	Not at all	No more than usual	Rather more than usual	Much more than usual	☐	☐	36
49.	**– been feeling unhappy and depressed?**	Not at all	No more than usual	Rather more than usual	Much more than usual	☐	☐	37
50.	**– been losing confidence in yourself?**	Not at all	No more than usual	Rather more than usual	Much more than usual	☐	☐	38
51.	**– been thinking of yourself as a worthless person?**	Not at all	No more than usual	Rather more than usual	Much more than usual	☐	☐	39
52.	**– felt that life is entirely hopeless?**	Not at all	No more than usual	Rather more than usual	Much more than usual	☐	☐	40
53.	**– been feeling hopeful about your own future?**	More so than usual	About same as usual	Less so than usual	Much less hopeful	☐	☐	41
54.	**– been feeling reasonably happy, all things considered?**	More so than usual	About same as usual	Less so than usual	Much less than usual	☐	☐	42

						Do not write in this space: Screening	Scoring	
55.	**– been feeling nervous and strung-up all the time?**	Not at all	No more than usual	Rather more than usual	Much more than usual	☐	☐	43
56.	**– felt that life isn't worth living?**	Not at all	No more than usual	Rather more than usual	Much more than usual	☐	☐	44
57.	**– thought of the possibility that you might make away with yourself?**	Definitely not	I don't think so	Has crossed my mind	Definitely have	☐	☐	45
58.	**– found at times you couldn't do anything because your nerves were too bad?**	Not at all	No more than usual	Rather more than usual	Much more than usual	☐	☐	46
59.	**– found yourself wishing you were dead and away from it all?**	Not at all	No more than usual	Rather more than usual	Much more than usual	☐	☐	47
60.	**– found that the idea of taking your own life kept coming into your mind?**	Definitely not	I don't think so	Has crossed my mind	Definitely has	☐	☐	48

The Effects of Benzodiazepines and Therapeutic Counselling in Different Populations

Interview No. 1

PRESENT STATE EXAMINATION

	Ø M B P 2 6 1 1	01-08
Section 1 – Identification Study Centre No.:		09-10
Name of Psychiatrist who Interviewed this Patient:	(leave blank)	11-12
	0 0 0	13-15
Patient's WHO Number:		16-18
Date of Interview:	Day Month Year	19-24
Time Taken for this Interview: in minutes		25-27

World Health Organization

The Effects of Benzodiazepines and Therapeutic Counselling in Different Populations

Interview No. 1

ØMBP2611

Section 2 – Present State Examination

Important Note

This score sheet should be used in conjunction with the PSE (9th edition) Interview Schedule.
Unless otherwise stated in the PSE Schedule the following codes should be used:

0 = Not present
1 = Moderate
2 = Severe
8 = Not known
9 = Not applicable

Time: Past 2 weeks

1. Introduction:

Patient's account of symptoms (see 140)

Reasons for inadequacy (tick as many as appropriate):

Denial or guardedness	☐	28
Incoherence	☐	29
Irrelevance	☐	30
Replies too brief	☐	31
Poverty of content of speech	☐	32
Inattention	☐	33
Refusal	☐	34
Patient mute, stuporous, etc.	☐	35
Other: ______	☐	36

.... *cut off* ....

2. Health, Worrying, Tension:

1.*	Subject's own subjective evaluation of present physical health	☐	37
2.	Presence of physical illness or handicap	☐	38
3.	Psychosomatic symptoms (special projects only)	☐	39
4.	Worrying	☐	40
5.	Tension pains	☐	41
6.	Tiredness or exhaustion	☐	42
7.	Muscular tension	☐	43
8.	Restlessness	☐	44
9.	Hypochondriasis	☐	45
10.	Subjective feeling of "nervous tension"	☐	46
11.	Hypersensitivity to noise	☐	47

3. Autonomic Anxiety:

11a.	Free-floating autonomic anxiety	☐	48
12.	Anxious foreboding with autonomic accompaniments	☐	49
13.	Autonomic anxiety due to delusions, etc.	☐	50

.... *cut off* ....

14.	Panic attacks with autonomic symptoms	☐	51
15.	Situational autonomic anxiety	☐	52
16.	Autonomic anxiety on meeting people	☐	53
17.	Specific phobias (not general situational anxiety)	☐	54
18.	Avoiding of anxiety provoking situations	☐	55

Detailed description of symptoms rated as present in items 1 – 18

World Health Organization

The Effects of Benzodiazepines and Therapeutic Counselling in Different Populations

Interview No. 1

ØMBP2611

Unless otherwise stated: 0 = Not present; 1 = Moderate; 2 = Severe; 8 = Not known; 9 = Not applicable

Section	No.	Item	Column
4. Thinking, Concentration, etc.:	19.	Subjectively inefficient thinking	56
	20.	Poor concentration	57
	21.	Neglect due to brooding	58
	22.	Loss of interest	59
		.... *cut off*	
5. Depressed Mood:	23.	Depressed mood	60
	24.	Hopelessness (subject's own view at present)	61
	25.	Suicidal plans or acts	62
		.... *cut off*	
	26.	Anxiety or depression primary	63
	27.	Morning depression	64
6. Self and Others:	28.	Social withdrawal	65
	29.	Self-depreciation	66
	30.	Lack of self-confidence with other people (in social relationships)	67
	31.	Simple ideas of reference (not delusions)	68
		.... *cut off*	
	32.	Guilty ideas of reference	69
	33.	Pathological guilt	70
7. Appetite, Sleep, Retardation, Libido:	34.	Loss of weight due to poor appetite	71
	35.	Delayed sleep	72
	36.	Subjective anergia and retardation	73
		.... *cut off*	
	37.	Early waking	74
	38.	Loss of libido (within present episode of illness and persisting during past month)	75
	39.	Premenstrual exacerbation	76
8. Irritability:	40.	Irritability	77
9. Expansive Mood and Ideation:	41.	Expansive mood (not ordinary high spirits)	78
	42.	Subjective ideomotor pressure	79
		.... *cut off*	
	43.	Grandiose ideas and actions	80
		Ø M B P 2 6 1 2	01-08
10. Obsessions:	44.	Obsessional checking and repeating	19
	45.	Obsessional cleanliness and similar rituals	20
	46.	Obsessional ideas and rumination	21

Detailed description of symptoms rated as present in items 19 – 46

World Health Organization

The Effects of Benzodiazepines and Therapeutic Counselling in Different Populations

Interview No. 1

0MBP2612

Unless otherwise stated: 0 = Not present, 1 = Moderate, 2 = Severe, 8 = Not known, 9 = Not applicable

11. Derealisation and Depersonalisation:	47.	Derealisation	☐	22
	48.	Depersonalisation	☐	23
12. Other Perceptual Disorders (not hallucinations):	49.	Delusional mood	☐	24
		.... *cut off*		
	50.	Heightened perception	☐	25
	51.	Dulled perception	☐	26
	52.	Changed perception	☐	27
	53.	Changed perception of time, including déjà vu	☐	28
	54.	Lost emotions	☐	29
13. Thought Reading, Insertion Echo, Broadcast:		.... *cut off*		
	55.	Thought insertion	☐	30
	56.	Thought broadcast	☐	31
	57.	Thought echo or commentary	☐	32
	58.	Thought block or withdrawal	☐	33
	59.	Delusions of thoughts being real	☐	34
14. Hallucinations:		.... *cut off*		
14A. Auditory Hallucinations:	60.	Non-verbal auditory hallucinations	☐	35
	61.	Verbal hallucinations based on depression or elation or voice calling subject	☐	36
	62.	Voice(s) discussion subject in third person or commenting on thoughts or actions (not based on depression or elation)	☐	37
	63.	Voice(s) speaking to subject (not based on depression or elation)	☐	38
	64.	Dissociative hallucinations (verbal and/or other)	☐	39
	65.	Pseudo- or true hallucinations	☐	40
14B. Visual Hallucinations:		.... *cut off*		
	66.	Visual hallucinations	☐	41
	67.	Delirious visual hallucinations	☐	42
14C. Other Hallucinations:		.... *cut off*		
	68.	Olfactory hallucinations	☐	43
	69.	Delusions that subject smells	☐	44
	70.	Other hallucinations and delusional elaboration	☐	45

Detailed description of symptoms rated as present in items 47 – 70

World Health Organization

The Effects of Benzodiazepines and Therapeutic Counselling in Different Populations

Interview No. 1

ØMBP2612

Unless otherwise stated: 0 = Not present, 1 = Moderate, 2 = Severe, 8 = Not known, 9 = Not applicable

15. Delusions: .... *cut off* ....

15A. Delusions of Control:	71.	Delusions of control	☐	46
15B. Misinterpretations, Misidentification and Delusions of Reference:	72.	Delusions of reference	☐	47
	73.	Delusional misinterpretation and misidentification	☐	48
15C. Delusions of Persecution:	74.	Delusions of persecution	☐	49
15D. Expansive Delusions:	75.	Delusions of assistance	☐	50
	76.	Delusions of grandiose abilities	☐	51
	77.	Delusions of grandiose identity	☐	52
15E. Delusions Concerning Various Types of Influence and Primary Delusions:	78.	Religious delusions	☐	53
	79.	Delusional explanations in terms of paranormal phenomena	☐	54
	80.	Delusional explanations in terms of physical forces	☐	55
	81.	Delusions of alien forces penetrating or controlling mind (or body)	☐	56
	82.	Primary delusions	☐	57
15F. Other Delusions:	83.	Subculturally influenced delusions	☐	58
	84.	Morbid jealousy	☐	59
	85.	Delusions of pregnancy	☐	60
	86.	Sexual delusions	☐	61
	87.	Fantastic delusions, delusional memories, delusional confabulations	☐	62
15G. Simple Delusions Based on Guilt, Depersonalisation, Hypochondriasis, etc.	88.	Delusions of guilt	☐	63
	89.	Simple delusions concerning appearance	☐	64
	90.	Delusions of depersonalisation	☐	65
	91.	Hypochondriacal delusions	☐	66
	92.	Delusions of catastrophe	☐	67
15H. General Ratings of Delutions and Hallucinations:	93.	Systematisation of delusions	☐	68
	94.	Evasiveness	☐	69
	95.	Preoccupation with delusions and hallucinations	☐	70
	96.	Acting out delusions	☐	71

Detailed description of symptoms rated as present in items 71 – 96

Unless otherwise stated: 0 = Not present, 1 = Moderate, 2 = Severe, 8 = Not known, 9 = Not applicable

16. Sensorium and Factors Affecting:	97. Fugues, blackouts, amnesia lasting more than one hour	☐	72
	98. Drug abuse during past month	☐	73
	99. Alcohol abuse during past month	☐	74
	100. Dissociative states during past month	☐	75
	101. Conversion symptoms	☐	76
	102. Clouding or stupor at examination	☐	77
	Any suspicion of poor memory or disorientation		
	103. Organic impairment of memory	☐	78
17. Insight:	104. If psychotic symtoms (sections 12–15)	☐	79
	105. If neurotic symptoms (sections 1–11 only)	☐	80
		Ø M B P 2 6 1 3	01-08
	106. Social impairment due to neurotic condition	☐	19
	107. Social impairment due to psychotic condition	☐	20
18.–20. Behaviour, Affect and Speech:			
Behaviour during Interview:	108. Self-neglect	☐	21
	109. Bizarre appearance	☐	22
	110. Slowness and underactivity	☐	23
	111. Agitation	☐	24
	112. Gross excitment and violence	☐	25
	113. Irreverent behaviour	☐	26
	114. Distractability	☐	27
	115. Embarrassing behaviour	☐	28
	116. Mannerisms and posturing	☐	29
	117. Stereotypies, etc.	☐	30
	118. Behaves as if hallucinated	☐	31
	119. Catatonic movements	☐	32
Affect during Interview:	120. Observed anxiety	☐	33
	121. Observed depression	☐	34
	122. Histrionic	☐	35
	123. Hypomanic affect	☐	36
	124. Hostile irritability	☐	37
	125. Suspicion	☐	38
	126. Perplexity (puzzlement)	☐	39
	127. Lability of mood	☐	40
	128. Blunted affect	☐	41
	129. Incongruity of affect	☐	42

Detailed description of symptoms rated as present in items 97 – 129

World Health Organization

The Effects of Benzodiazepines and Therapeutic Counselling in Different Populations

Interview No. 1

ØMBP2613

Unless otherwise stated: 0 = Not present, 1 = Moderate, 2 = Severe, 8 = Not known, 9 = Not applicable

Speech during Interview:

130.	Slow speech	☐	43
131.	Pressure of speech	☐	44
132.	Non-social speech	☐	45
133.	Muteness	☐	46
134.	Restricted quantity of speech	☐	47
135.	Neologisms and idiosyncratic use of words or phrases	☐	48
136.	Incoherence of speech	☐	49
137.	Flight of ideas	☐	50
138.	Poverty of content of speech	☐	51
139.	Misleading answers	☐	52
140.	Re-rate adequacy of interview	☐	53

State Overall Diagnosis According to Terminology Used at Your Centre:

____

____

______________________________ ☐☐☐☐ (leave blank) 54-57

Diagnosis Classification:

How would you classify your diagnosis according to the Ninth Revision of the International Classification of Diseases?

Use as many codes as necessary, start with first, most important diagnosis.

Write ICD code number in the boxes

1.	☐☐☐.☐	58-61
2.	☐☐☐.☐	62-65
3.	☐☐☐.☐	66-69
4.	☐☐☐.☐	70-73
5.	☐☐☐.☐	74-77

Detailed description of symptoms rated as present in items 130 – 140

World Health Organization

The Effects of Benzodiazepines and Therapeutic Counselling in Different Populations

Interview No. 1

RATING SCALE FOR SIDE EFFECTS

Introductory Note

This schedule is composed of two sections: Section 1 covers basic data necessary for the identification of the patient, Section 2 lists a series of rating scales for the side effects presumed due to the drugs.

In Section 2 the rater should enquire systematically for each symptom and enter the appropriate code number into each box.

Ø M B P 2 3 1 1 01-08

Section 1 – Identification

Study Centre No.: ☐☐ 09-10

Name of Researcher who Interviewed this Patient: ____________ ☐☐ (leave blank) 11-12

0 0 0 13-15

Patient's WHO Number: ☐☐☐ 16-18

Date of Interview: Day Month Year ☐☐☐☐☐☐ 19-24

Section 2 – Rating Scale for Side Effects 0 25

Physical Tiredness:
0 = None
1 = Slightly tired, but needs no extra rest
2 = Has to lie down and rest at times or very tired but unable to rest
3 = Lies all day
☐ 0 26-27

Dizziness:
0 = None
1 = Occasional slight dizziness
2 = Constantly slightly dizzy, or occasional severe dizziness
3 = Constant severe dizziness; has to lie down
☐ 0 28-29

Dizziness on Getting up Suddenly:
0 = None
1 = Feels slightly like fainting on sudden raising
2 = Has to rise slowly to avoid feeling like fainting
3 = Fainting frequently independing of position
☐ 0 30-31

Dryness of Mouth:
0 = None
1 = Some, but not subjectively disturbing
2 = Obvious, but not severe or painful
3 = Severe, makes speaking difficult
☐ 0 32-33

Drowsiness:
0 = None
1 = Slight
2 = Moderate, some interference
3 = Severe, interference to daily routine marked
☐ 0 34-35

Interference with Sexual Functioning: (if applicable)
0 = None
1 = Slight impairment
2 = Moderate impairment
3 = Severe impairment
☐ 0 36-37

Other Symptoms Considered during Interview to be Important: (specify)
1 = Slight impairment
2 = Moderate impairment
3 = Severe impairment

A. ____________ ☐ 0 38-39

B. ____________ ☐ 0 40-41

C. ____________ ☐

GENERAL PRACTITIONER'S RATING – NEED-FOR-TREATMENT SCALES

Section 1 – Identification

Ø M B P 2 2 0 1 01-08

Study Centre No.:
02 = Bombay
08 = Ibadan
09 = London
10 = Tokyo
☐☐ 09-10

Name of Researcher who Interviewed this Patient: ____________ ☐☐ (leave blank) 11-12

Patient's Registration Number in Facility: ____________ 0 0 0 13-15

Patient's WHO Number: To be filled in later by investigator if patient is definitely included ☐☐☐ 16-18

Date of Interview: Day Month Year ☐☐☐☐☐☐ 19-24

Section 2 – Need-for-Treatment Scales

1. Type of Compaint:
1 = *No complaint (exclusion category)*
2 = *Complaints are physical in origin, emotional factors of no importance (exclusion category)*
3 = Worries or emotional factors presented but not necessarily relevant to the patient's complaint, but intervention not indicated
4 = Needs anti-anxiety agent or some counselling – general practitioner able to deal with
☐ 25

2. Psychiatric Severity of Complaint:
1 = Normal
2 = Such complaints as he/she has do not merit psychiatric help
3 = Needs some psychiatric help, but outpatient treatment is satisfactory
4 = *Moderately ill, inpatient treatment probably would help (exclusion category)*
5 = *Severely ill, admission to hospital is essential (exclusion category)*
☐ 26

3. If I Were Treating the Patient I Would Recommend:
1 = No treatment
2 = Counselling only
3 = An anti-anxiety agent such as Valium
4 = *A strong medication such as an anti-depressant or phenothiazine (exclusion category)*
5 = *Admission to hospital (exclusion category)*
☐ 27

If the reply to **any one** of the items 1, 2 or 3 above is in the *EXCLUSION CATEGORY*, exclude patient.

Code:
0 = PATIENT EXCLUDED
1 = SCREENING INTERVIEW CONTINUED
☐ 28

If patient EXCLUDED: **Please keep these forms for subsequent return to WHO in Geneva**

World Health Organization

The Effects of Benzodiazepines and Therapeutic Counselling in Different Populations

Screening Interview

ØMBP2201

Section 3 – Further Information

0 = No
1 = *Yes*

1. Does the Patient Live Too Far Away to be Followed Up at Home? ☐ 29

2. Is the Patient Physically Ill to a Point that will Interfere with His/Her Social or Emotional Function or State? (e.g. malaria, amoebiasis, influenza, pregnancy, etc.) ☐ 30

If yes, please specify: ______

3. Is the Patient Unwilling to Come Back in 2, 6 and 12 Weeks for Follow-up (given a final visit inducement)? ☐ 31

4. Is the Patient Already on Psychotropic Medication? (anxiolytics, antidepressants, neuroleptics or opiates) ☐ 32

If yes, please specify: ______

5. Is Alcoholism or Drug Dependence a Problem? ☐ 33

If the reply to **any one** of the items 1–5 above is *YES*, exclude patient.

Code: **0 = PATIENT EXCLUDED**
1 = SCREENING INTERVIEW CONTINUED ☐ 34

If patient EXCLUDED: **Please keep these forms for subsequent return to WHO in Geneva**

If screening interview CONTINUED: **Please complete this form and refer the patient to the investigator for further interview**

Patient's First Name: ______

Patient's surname (optional): ______

Date of Birth / Age in Years: Estimate if necessary or fill in 9s if unknown, e.g.. Day Month Year Age (yrs) 9 9 0 1 4 1 3 7 — Day Month Year Age (yrs) ☐☐☐☐☐☐ ☐☐ 35-42

Sex: 1 = Male 4 = Female ☐ 43

Marital Status: Rate for majority of time in last 6 months

1 = Single
2 = Married
3 = Divorced
4 = Separated
5 = Widowed
6 = Common law marriage, consensual union, cohabiting
7 = Other (specify: ______)
9 = Unknown

☐ 44

Patient's Permanent Address: ______

Any other address through which patient can be traced? ______

Name and Address of Key Informant about Patient: ______

Relationship to patient: ______

DEMOGRAPHIC DESCRIPTION

ØMBP2111 01-08

Section 1 — Identification

Study Centre No.: ☐☐ 09-10

Name of Researcher who Interviewed this Patient: ______ ☐☐ (leave blank) 11-12

:0:0:0: 13-15

Patient's WHO Number: ☐☐☐ 16-18

Date of Interview: Day Month Year ☐☐☐☐☐☐ 19-24

Section 2 — General Information

Date of Birth / Age in Years: Estimate if necessary or fill in "9"s if unknown (e.g. 990141 37) Day Month Year ☐☐☐☐☐☐ Age (yrs) ☐☐ 25-32

Sex: 1 = Male 4 = Female ☐ 33

Ethnic Group as Stated by Patient: ______ ☐☐ (leave blank) 34-35

Is the Person Interviewed a Member of a Minority Group? (use judgment)
0 = No
1 = Yes
9 = Impossible to judge
☐ 36

If yes, please specify: ______

Patient's Current Residence:
1 = Rural
2 = Urban - peripheral
3 = Urban - central
4 = Other (specify: ______)
9 = Unknown
☐ 37

How long has patient lived in the present place? Estimate number of years ☐☐ 38-39

Type of Household:
1 = Nuclear (no more than one two generation set)
2 = Extended vertically (one three generation set)
3 = Extended horizontally (two or more two generation sets)
4 = Extended both ways (one or more three generation sets, and one or more one or two generation sets; or two or more three generation sets)
9 = Impossible to assess
☐ 40

Number of household members: 99 = Unknown 01 = Patient lives alone ☐☐ 41-42

Number of children living with patient: 99 = Unknown ☐☐ 43-44

Number of children under 5 years old living with patient: 99 = Unknown ☐☐ 45-46

Are the patient's current housing conditions unsatisfactory in any way?
0 = No
1 = Yes
9 = Uncertain
☐ 47

If yes, please specify: ______

Rate Socioeconomic Status of Household on 5 Point Scale: (use judgment)
1 = Lowest
2 = Below average
3 = Average
4 = Above average
5 = Highest
9 = Can't estimate
☐ 48

Highest Level of Education that Patient Reached:

0 = Illiterate
1 = Never at school, literate
2 = Less than 5 completed years at school
3 = 5–12 completed years of school
4 = More than 12 completed years but did not complete university
5 = University graduate
6 = Postgraduate education completed
7 = Vocational education
8 = Other (specify: ______________________)
9 = Unknown

☐ 49

What is the Current Main Occupation of the Patient?

Describe what he/she actually does; if subject has more than one occupation describe the source of highest earned personal income:

____

____

____

☐☐☐ (leave blank) 50-52

What is the Patient's Current Working Status?

2 = Self employed
3 = Employed
4 = Unemployed
5 = On sick leave, currently employed
6 = On sickness (disablement, unemployed)
7 = Other (specify: ______________________)
8 = Not applicable (e.g. student, housewife, pensioner)

☐ 53

If gainfully employed: Complete next box with "8" and continue with the question following afterwards

If not gainfully employed, give reason for unemployment:

0 = Student
1 = Housewife
2 = Old age pensioner
3 = Has other income (excluding pension, social welfare)
4 = Because of general unemployment
5 = Because of illness, or disability (specify which: ______________________)
6 = Work as unpaid worker in family concern
7 = Other reasons (specify: ______________________)
9 = Unknown

☐ 54

If not gainfully employed: Complete next box with "8" and continue with the question following afterwards

If gainfully employed:
Does he/she work full-time or part-time? (regardless of whether patient has more than one job)

0 = Full-time
1 = Part-time
2 = Other arrangements (specify: ______________________)
9 = Unknown

☐ 55

Section 3 – Physical and Mental Health

Has the Patient had Serious Physical Illness or Disability in the Past?

0 = No
1 = Yes (specify: ______________________)
9 = Uncertain

☐ 56

☐☐☐ (leave blank) 57-59

Has the Patient ever had Treatment for Mental Illness, or is there Evidence of Untreated Serious Mental Illness before this Treatment Phase?

0 = Neither
1 = Outpatient treatment (where? ______________________)
2 = Inpatient treatment (where? ______________________)
3 = Outpatient and inpatient treatment (where? ______________________)
4 = Other treatment (e.g. traditional practices, etc.) (specify: ______________________)
5 = No treatment but evidence of untreated mental illness
9 = Unknown

☐ 60

If patient gives history of treatment for mental illness:
What was the reason for treatment? (give diagnosis if available) ________ ☐☐☐ (leave blank) 61-63

When was the Last Time the Patient saw a Physican? How many months ago? ☐☐ 64-65

Section 4 — Diagnosis and Classification

State Diagnosis According to your own Practice:

____

____

________ ☐☐☐☐ (leave blank) 66-69

Diagnosis Classification:

How would you classify your diagnosis according to the Ninth Revision of the International Classification of Diseases?

Use as many codes as necessary; start with the first most important diagnosis. Write ICD code number in the boxes,

e.g.: Anxiety states = 300.0 = 3 0 0 . 0

☐☐☐.☐ 70-73

☐☐☐.☐ 74-77

Information which could not be Coded but which you Consider Important in this Case:

____

____

____

____

____

____

BRIEF LIFE EVENTS QUESTIONNAIRE

Introductory Note

This schedule is intended to rate the occurrence of events in the past three months which may have affected the patient. The interviewer should seek by question and cross examination to determine the following about each item:

1. Did the event occur? If so, describe where indicated.
2. If so, when – timing within the passing three months is especially critical, count from the date of interview.
3. Was the event independent of the patient's action – i.e., could not have occurred as a result of anything the patient did in past three months, or as a result of his/her present condition. Rate "1" for such independent events (e.g., patient's place of work shut down). This rating is for events independent of anything the patient could have done.
4. Was the event probably provoked by the patient's action, i.e., unlikely to have happened without the patient's actions. Rate "2" for dependent events (e.g., patient's girlfriend left him because of his persistent irritable mood).
5. Uncertain whether event is independent of patient's behaviour or not. If the event may be due to the patient's action, but this is uncertain, rate "3" (e.g., if patient moved after purchasing a house four months previously).

Thus, a rating of

- "1" is for events totally independent of the patient's action
- "2" is for events probably resulting from the patient's action
- "3" is for events where there is uncertainty if they were a result of the patient's action or not

Any event which occurs should only be rated once. Rate in most relevant section. | Ø | M | B | P | 2 | 4 | 3 | 1 | 01-08

Section 1 – Identification

Study Centre No.: [ ][ ] 09-10

Name of Researcher who Interviewed this Patient: [ ] [ ][ ] (leave blank) 11-12

:0:0:0: 13-15

Patient's WHO Number: [ ][ ][ ] 16-18

Date of Interview: Day [ ][ ] Month [ ][ ] Year [ ][ ] 19-24

Section 2 – Life Events

Rating scales:

Time of Onset

Rate as accurately as possible time between event onset and present interview as follows:

0 = Event not occurred
1 = Within 1 month
2 = Within 2 months
3 = Within 3 months
4 = Within 4–6 months
5 = Within 7–9 months
6 = Within 10–12 months
7 = More than 12 months, less than 2 years if problem still present

Independence of Event

0 = Event did not occur
1 = Probably independent (not due to patient's action)
2 = Probably dependent (due to patient's action)
3 = Uncertain whether due to patient or not
9 = Insufficient information

Have any of the following occurred in the patient's life in the past three months?

		Time since Onset of Event	Independence of Event	
Illness or Injury:	**Probe:** Have you or anyone in the family had a serious illness or injury in the last 3 months, this is in – / – / – / – (mention last 4 months). Has anyone died or is this likely in the near future? Anyone attempted suicide? Accidents or illness in children, close friends (specify how serious is the event)? When did this occur?			
1. Physical illness or injury to patient? (e.g., sufficient to require medical treatment and bedrest over a week)	Specify: ______	☐	☐	25-26
2. Physical illness or injury to members of family* or close friend**:	Specify: ______	☐	☐	27-28
3. Death or impending death of a close relative (if not rated above) – spouse, parent, child, sibling – or other significant person?	Specify: ______	☐	☐	29-30
4. Patient had an accident:	Specify and indicate extent of injury: ______	☐	☐	31-32
5. Patient, close relative or friend attempted suicide:	Specify: ______	☐	☐	33-34
Schooling:	**Probe:** Has there been anything important happened in your schooling? Starting, finishing, failing examinations, etc. When?			
6. Change in schooling or education (changed, finished or started school or university, failed important exams):	Specify: ______	☐	☐	35-36

* Relatives emotionally important to patient

** Non-relatives emotionally important to patient

World Health Organization

The Effects of Benzodiazepines and Therapeutic Counselling in Different Populations

Interview No. 3

ØMBP2431

Time of Onset
Rate as accurately as possible time between event onset and present interview as follows:
0 = Event not occurred
1 = Within 1 month
2 = Within 2 months
3 = Within 3 months
4 = Within 4–6 months
5 = Within 7–9 months
6 = Within 10–12 months
7 = More than 12 months, less than 2 years if problem still present

Independence of Event
0 = Event did not appear
1 = Probably independent (not due to patient's action)
2 = Probably dependen (due to patient's action)
3 = Uncertain whether due to patient or not
9 = Insufficient information

		Time since Onset of Event	Independence of Event	
Work:	**Probe:** Are you working? If not, how long have you been out of work? Have there been any important changes at work, where you work? What was this due to? When?			
7. Major change of work (e.g., new type of location of work, marked change in work hours, or responsibilities, promotion, demotion):	Specify:	☐	☐	37-38
8. Stopped working, left, dismissed or retired:	Specify:	☐	☐	39-40
Financial:	**Probe:** Has your income or that of a close relative gone down recently? Any other money problems? Any loss or theft in past 4 months? When?			
9. A material / financial loss or difficulty (include if there has been a significant or lasting reduction or increase in personal or household income; a major theft; or loss or damage of important personal property):	Specify:	☐	☐	41-42
10. Legal troubles affecting the patient or close relative:	Specify:	☐	☐	43-44
Relationship:	**Probe:** Have you or anyone close to you got married in past 4 months – / – / – / – (i.e., name them), or anyone separated or divorced? Have any important or close relationships broken up? When?			
11. Patient married:	Specify:	☐	☐	45-46
12. A divorce or lasting separation from spouse or sexual partner:	Specify:	☐	☐	47-48
13. A major change in relationship with spouse or sexual partner, not including divorce or separation:	Specify:	☐	☐	49-50
14. A major change in a significant personal relationship (other than rated in 12 or 13), not included above:	Specify:	☐	☐	51-52

The Effects of Benzodiazepines and Therapeutic Counselling in Different Populations

Interview No. 3

ØMBP2431

Time of Onset
Rate as accurately as possible time between event onset and present interview as follows:
0 = Event not occurred
1 = Within 1 month
2 = Within 2 months
3 = Within 3 months
4 = Within 4–6 months
5 = Within 7–9 months
6 = Within 10–12 months
7 = More than 12 months, less than 2 years if problem still present

Independence of Event
0 = Event did not appear
1 = Probably independent (not due to patient's action)
2 = Probably dependent (due to patient's action)
3 = Uncertain whether due to patient or not
9 = Insufficient information

Time since Onset of Event | **Independence of Event**

Children and Family:

Probe: Have any children been born to you or your family? Are you (or is your wife or consensual partner) pregnant? Did anyone have a miscarriage or abortion? When?

15. A child was born to the patient (if pregnancy began before any sign of malaise, rate as independent): Specify: ______ ☐ ☐ 53-54

16. Pregnancy, miscarriage, abortion or still-birth (experienced by patient if female, or by wife or girlfriend of patient, if male). Infertility if and when recognized as a problem: Specify: ______ ☐ ☐ 55-56

Probe: Has there been any big change in the family in the past 4 months? When? Anyone come to stay or moved away? Have you moved residence recently?

17. A major change in family structure (affecting family as a whole, e.g. splitting of family, children leave home, relatives move in, etc.): Specify: ______ ☐ ☐ 57-58

Other Changes, Losses:

Probe: Can you think of any other big changes in your life which I have not asked about? Any important losses or disappointments which have not been mentioned?

18. Change of residence by patient to a near or far location (move house): Specify: ______ ☐ ☐ 59-60

19. Other significant event changes in the pattern of patient's day to day life: Specify: ______ ☐ ☐ 61-62

20. Other significant losses not mentioned: Specify: ______ ☐ ☐ 63-64

Probe: Has there been any other change which might be worrying – for example, a change in tax or a curfew? (Rather use own knowledge and question patient on importance of known social changes, whether they affect patient.)

21. Any major change or anticipated social changes due to politcal, legal or other reasons, e.g., change in form of government, imposition of martial law, war, or uprooting not included above: Specify: ______ ☐ ☐ 65-66

IMPORTANT Please remember to put this cardboard between the form to be completed (together with its copy) and the following one. This prevents copying of your entries onto several forms.

World Health Organization

The Effects of Benzodiazepines and Therapeutic Counselling in Different Populations

Ø M B F

PERSONAL TREATMENT RECORD

Patient's Name:

Patient's Registration No. in Facility:

Patient's WHO Number:

Name of Researcher who Filled in this Form:

Study Centre No.:
02 = Bombay 09 = London
08 = Ibadan 10 = Tokyo

Day Mo

Date of First Contact:

Date Medication Started:

	Trial Treatment Day	Dosage Prescribed (tabs given)	Tablets Taken	Other Treatment Describe (If Counselling was given: Please indicate and give date and time spent for each session)	Day	Dosage	Reason for Clinical Deci
	1				1		
	2				2		
	3				3		
WEEK 1	4				4		
	5				5		
	6				6		
	7				7		
	8				8		
	9				9		
	10				10		
WEEK 2	11				11		
	12				12		
	13				13		
	14				14		
	15				15		
	16				16		
	17				17		
WEEK 3	18				18		
	19				19		
	20				20		
	21				21		
	22				22		
	23				23		
	24				24		
WEEK 4	25				25		
	26				26		
	27				27		
	28				28		
	29				29		
	30				30		
	31				31		
WEEK 5	32				32		
	33				33		
	34				34		
	35				35		

IMPORTANT Please remember to put this cardboard between the form to be completed (together with its copy) and the following one. This prevents copying of your entries onto several forms.

World Health Organization

The Effects of Benzodiazepines and Therapeutic Counselling in Different Populations

Personal Treatment
(continued)

ØMBP2801

	Trial Treatment Day	Dosage Prescribed (tabs given)	Tablets Taken	Other Treatment Describe (If Counselling was given: Please indicate and give date and time spent for each session)	Day	Dosage	Reason for Clinical Decisio
	36				36		
	37				37		
	38				38		
WEEK 6	39				39		
	40				40		
	41				41		
	42				42		
	43				43		
	44				44		
	45				45		
WEEK 7	46				46		
	47				47		
	48				48		
	49				49		
	50				50		
	51				51		
	52				52		
WEEK 8	53				53		
	54				54		
	55				55		
	56				56		
	57				57		
	58				58		
	59				59		
WEEK 9	60				60		
	61				61		
	62				62		
	63				63		
	64				64		
	65				65		
	66				66		
WEEK 10	67				67		
	68				68		
	69				69		
	70				70		
	71				71		
	72				72		
	73				73		
WEEK 11	74				74		
	75				75		
	76				76		
	77				77		
	78				78		
	79				79		
	80				80		
WEEK 12	81				81		
	82				82		
	83				83		

World Health Organization

The Effects of Benzodiazepines and Therapeutic Counselling in Different Populations

Audit of Counselling

A Introduction

The ratings in this schedule are intended to determine what the patient is being counselled about, how the counsellor conducts the sessions technically and what the counsellor feels is most important, as well as progress the counsellor feels has been made.

The schedule is composed of two parts:

- Part A: Quantitative Description of Interview is to be filled in immediately after each counselling session.
  This part consists of four sections:
  Section 1 – covers basic data necessary for the identification of the patient.
  Section 2 – a rating scale to determine what subjects were dealt with in the session. The investigator should estimate the percentage of time he/she spent on any of these particular problems.
  Section 3 – the technique used by the counsellor and its importance within the interview. The investigator should use his/her best estimate of the importance and percentage of time he/she spent using a particular technique.
  Section 4 – the investigator should use his/her objective judgement to assess the quality of client/counsellor interaction to identify how the patient reacted within each counselling session.

- Part B: Final Audit of Counselling and Retrospective Assessment of Change is to be filled in when the patient's counselling treatment has been completed. Include if counselling consisted of two or more sessions, either when counselling has finished or the patient has dropped out.
  This part consists of three sections:
  Section 1 – the identification of the patient.
  Section 2 – covers the importance and progress achieved for each problem area which may have been discussed during the interview. The counsellor rates his/her judgement of the overall importance of any problem area leading to the patient's distress. Progress is divided into Objective Change consisting of the counsellor's rating of actual changes in the patient's circumstances, e.g. improved housing conditions, reduced number of arguments with spouse, etc., and Subjective Change consisting of changes in the way the patient feels about the problem(s), e.g. housing or sexual problems may or may not have been improved but the patient may nevertheless feel better or worse about it.
  Section 3 – the counsellor's overall evaluation of the patient's improvement and the contribution of counselling to it.

B Definition of Terms Used

1.	Money	Include any difficulties arising out of shortage of money for food or essentials for self or family. Debts, bills, rent arrears, etc.
2.	Housing	Include homelessness, facing eviction, overcrowded, too large to be manageable, tenant problems, vandalism, any bad living conditions, e.g. undone repairs.
3.	Work	Include difficulties or disappointments/dislike of work, colleagues, superiors or conditions. Inability to cope. Unemployment, redundancy, retirement, etc.
4.	School / study	Include exam strain or failure. Difficulties with teacher. Disappointments in relation to the nature of the work/performance. Illiteracy. Concern about a relation's schooling. School phobia. Truancy.

5.	Legal problems	Include all problems arising out of legal affairs, civil/criminal. Exclude divorce.
6.	Child care	Include lack of emotion for child/children. Feelings of violence towards child/children. Sibling rivalry/jealousy. Lack of confidence in dealing with child. Inability to control/discipline. Difficulty with handling. Exclude legal matters such as custody by State (under Legal) or custody in relation to divorce (under Divorce).
7.	Loneliness	Include social isolation. Lack of friends/acquaintances, inability to confide in others.
8.	Illness / health	Include headaches, backache, pain from injury, operation. Exclude pregnancy (under Pregnancy). Include worries in relation to possible or known illness.
9.	Bereavement	Include sadness, worry or depression in relation to death. Include animals.
10.	Pregnancy	Include fear of birth, discomfort, worry regarding abnormality, race or sex of child. Spontaneous miscarriage, difficult birth. Ectopic pregnancy. Exclude abortion, i.e. wilful termination of pregnancy.
11.	Abortion	Include wilful termination of pregnancy, self-induced/by hospital/nursing home/abortionist. Guilt regarding present or past abortion. Worry regarding abortion procedure. Religious conflicts regarding decision, etc.
12.	Family planning	Include fear of pregnancy, distaste regarding method of contraception. Worry about efficacy of method of contraception. Conflict with partner re method or acceptability of contraception.
13.	Sexual problems	Include difficulties in sexual functioning or disappointment with regard to sex. Sexual deviancy.
14.	Love relationships	Where focus is on difficulty in relationships, rate here. If principle difficulty arises out of a more specific problem, rate where appropriate. Include material conflicts here. Rate divorce/separation difficulties under 17. Rate sexual problems above (13).
15.	Family relationships	Rate problems with relatives other than spouse such as lack of understanding, rows, conflicts over responsibilities and duties or burden resulting from a relative's own problem. Rate parental control and difficulties rearing children under item 6, Child Care.
16.	Social relationships	Rate problems not involving a love partner or relative such as conflicts with neighbours or friends, difficulties meeting people or forming relationships should be rated under item 7, Loneliness.
17.	Divorce / separation	Include any problem arising out of separation/divorce, e.g. arguments, custody decisions regarding money, bribery, alimony. Problems arising out of the marital home, problems over management of children.
18.	Gambling	Include all problems arising out of gambling, e.g. money difficulties, disharmony, lies. Exclude legal consequence (under Legal).
19.	Alcoholism	Include any difficulties arising out of heavy drinking. Include marital/sexual problems.
20.	Religion	Include all problems arising out of religious conflict, disharmony, e.g. mixed religion marriages, etc.
21.	Racial / cultural	Include any problem arising out of this, i.e. mixed marriage, neighbourhood disharmony, involving tension or difficulties related to ethnic, cultural, tribal disharmony at either a personal or community level. (Do not rate same item in two places.)
22.	Drug abuse	Include any difficulties or worries regarding drugs, i.e. cannabis, L.S.D., etc. Addiction, overdose, etc.
23.	Self doubt / lack of confidence	Include any problem relating to lack of confidence, self-deprecation.
24.	Abnormal fears	Include here any worry regarding fears or thoughts where there is little or no evidence of the problem existing, e.g. cancer phobia, etc.
25.	Other	Include here any problem area not mentioned in above categories.

AUDIT OF COUNSELLING – PART A

Quantitative Description of the Interview ØMBP2911 01-08

Section 1 – Identification

Study Centre No.: ☐☐ 09-10

Name of Researcher who Interviewed this Patient: ____________ ☐☐ (leave blank) 11-12

0:0:0: 13-15

Patient's Registration Number in Facility: ____________

Patient's WHO Number: ☐☐☐ 16-18

Date of Interview: Day ☐☐ Month ☐☐ Year ☐☐ 19-24

Total Time Spent for this Interview: in minutes ☐☐☐ 25-27

Time Spent in General Conversation: in minutes ☐☐☐ 28-30

Section 2 – Present Problems

Estimate the percentage of time spent on any particular problem. If 99 or 100 % rate "99". For any of the items rated please give details on the following page.

1.	Money:	☐☐	31-32
2.	Housing:	☐☐	33-34
3.	Work:	☐☐	35-36
4.	School / study:	☐☐	37-38
5.	Legal problems:	☐☐	39-40
6.	Child care:	☐☐	41-42
7.	Loneliness:	☐☐	43-44
8.	Illness / health:	☐☐	45-46
9.	Bereavement:	☐☐	47-48
10.	Pregnancy:	☐☐	49-50
11.	Abortion:	☐☐	51-52
12.	Family planning:	☐☐	53-54
13.	Sexual problems:	☐☐	55-56
14.	Love or sexual relationships:	☐☐	57-58
15.	Family relationships:	☐☐	59-60
16.	Social relationships:	☐☐	61-62
17	Divorce / separation:	☐☐	63-64
18.	Gambling:	☐☐	65-66
19.	Alcoholism:	☐☐	67-68
20.	Religion:	☐☐	69-70
21.	Racial / cultural:	☐☐	71-72
22.	Drug abuse:	☐☐	73-74
23.	Self doubt / lack of confidence:	☐☐	75-76

Detailed description of items rated on page 1

World Health Organization

The Effects of Benzodiazepines and Therapeutic Counselling in Different Populations

Audit of Counselling – Part A (1)

Ø	M	B	P	2	9	1	2	01-08

Section 3 – Techniques Used by Counsellor During Interview

To your best estimate, rate the percentage of time spent on any particular technique and its importance within the interview.

Rate importance as follows:

0 = Did not take place
1 = Occurred but of little or no value
2 = Of some or substantial value
3 = Most important intervention

	Technique	Description	Percentage of Time	Importance	
1.	History taking or questioning:	Specific questions to gain optimum information on present problems.	⊔⊔	⊔	19-21
2.	Exploration:	Further questioning to focus interview, clarify the client's and counsellor's thoughts to arrive at a better understanding of the problem.	⊔⊔	⊔	22-24
3.	Permitting silence:	Purposely allowing silence which is initiated by the patient.	⊔⊔	⊔	25-27
4.	Ventilation:	Allowing the patient to take the initiative and talk or express feelings at some length when obtaining information is not the main motive.	⊔⊔	⊔	28-30
5.	Encouragement/reinforcement:	An effort by the counsellor to positively endorse/reinforce or encourage.	⊔⊔	⊔	31-33
6.	Advice giving:	Offering advice about dealing with practical issues or offering suggestions, alternatives, etc.	⊔⊔	⊔	34-36
7.	Interpretation / insights giving:	Helping the patient to understand why the problem is occurring by looking at it from a less subjective viewpoint. Include any attempt to re-interpret the patient's thoughts, feelings, fantasies or actions in a different conceptual frame-work.	⊔⊔	⊔	37-39
8.	Challenging:	Deliberately making an assertion which might be contrary to what the patient expects or wants in order to produce a re-action or response in the patient which would facilitate a change in attitude or practice, e.g., suggesting to the patient that he is using his illness to gain sympathy or to manipulate others.	⊔⊔	⊔	40-42

Section 4 – Quality of Client/Counsellor Relationship

Make an objective judgement to assess the relationship between the client and the counsellor.

Rate type of relationship as follows:

0 = Not present
1 = Present at times
2 = Present throughout interview
9 = Uncertain

	Relationship	Description	Rating	
1.	Acceptance:	Willingness on part of patient to accept this form of help. Patient's willingness to participate in the session indicates co-operation.	⊔	43
2.	Empathy:	The counsellor feels he/she understands patient's feelings, conflicts or problems.	⊔	44
3.	Evasiveness:	Patient is reluctant to focus on issue raised by counsellor and evades any or most important issues.	⊔	45
4.	Hostility:	Patient appears to dislike or finds unacceptable the ideas of counselling or appears to be hypersensitive or embarrassed by probing certain issues raised during session. Also rate if patient seems hostile though reason is unclear.	⊔	46

Remarks:

The Effects of Benzodiazepines and Therapeutic Counselling in Different Populations

AUDIT OF COUNSELLING – PART B

Final Audit of Counselling and Retrospective Assessment of Change | Ø | M | B | P | 2 | 9 | 0 | 1 | 01-08

Section 1 – Identification

Study Centre No.: [ ][ ] 09-10

Name of Researcher who Interviewed this Patient: [ ] [ ][ ] (leave blank) 11-12

:0:0:0: 13-15

Patient's Registration Number in Facility: [ ]

Patient's WHO Number: [ ][ ][ ] 16-18

Date this Schedule was filled in: Day Month Year [ ][ ][ ][ ][ ][ ] 19-24

Section 2 – Importance and Progress

This section consists of 3 ratings:

– **Importance:** The counsellor's best judgment of the overall importance of any of the patient's problems

– **Objective Change:** To rate material or identifiable progress in terms of event which actually occurred

– **Subjective Change:** The counsellor should use his/her objective judgment to assess changes in the way the patient feels about the problems

Rating scales

Importance	Objective Change	Subjective Change
0 = Nil	0 = Same – no change specifiable	0 = Same – no change specifiable
1 = Arose in interview, of little overall consequence	1 = Worse – deterioration must be specifiable	1 = Worse – patient expresses increased concern, worry, despair
2 = One of several issues causing patient distress	2 = Minimal – change can be specified but is minor	2 = Slight to moderate – some decrease in distress expressed by patient
3 = Very important, not outweighing all other issues	3 = Substantial – significant improvement but some difficulty remains	3 = Marked improvement – no longer causing distress but still not totally resolved
4 = Most important, grossly outweighing all other issues	4 = Complete resolution of problems	4 = Complete resolution – problem no longer of any concern
8 = Not applicable	8 = Not applicable	8 = Not applicable

	Importance	Objective Change	Subjective Change	
1. Money:	[ ]	[ ]	[ ]	25-27
2. Housing:	[ ]	[ ]	[ ]	28-30
3. Work:	[ ]	[ ]	[ ]	31-33
4. School / study:	[ ]	[ ]	[ ]	34-36
5. Legal problems:	[ ]	[ ]	[ ]	37-39
6. Child care:	[ ]	[ ]	[ ]	40-42

World Health Organization

The Effects of Benzodiazepines and Therapeutic Counselling in Different Populations

Audit of Counselling – Part B

0MBP2901

Importance
0 = Nil
1 = Arose in interview, of little overall consequence
2 = One of several issues causing patient distress
3 = Very important, not outweighing all other issues
4 = Most important, grossly outweighing all other issues
8 = Not applicable

Objective Change
0 = Same – no change specifiable
1 = Worse – deterioration must be specifiable
2 = Minimal – change can be specified but is minor
3 = Substantial – significant improvement but some difficulty remains
4 = Complete resolution of problems
8 = Not applicable

Subjective Change
0 = Same – no change specifiable
1 = Worse – patient expresses increased concern, worry, despair
2 = Slight to moderate – some decrease in distress expressed by patient
3 = Marked improvement – no longer causing distress but still not totally resolved
4 = Complete resolution – problem no longer of any concern
8 = Not applicable

		Importance	**Objective Change**	**Subjective Change**	
7.	Loneliness:	☐	☐	☐	43-45
8.	Illness / health:	☐	☐	☐	46-48
9.	Bereavement:	☐	☐	☐	49-51
10.	Pregnancy:	☐	☐	☐	52-54
11.	Abortion:	☐	☐	☐	55-57
12.	Family planning:	☐	☐	☐	58-60
13.	Sexual problems:	☐	☐	☐	61-63
14.	Love and sexual relationships:	☐	☐	☐	64-66
15.	Family relationships:	☐	☐	☐	67-69
16.	Social relationships:	☐	☐	☐	70-72
17.	Divorce / separation:	☐	☐	☐	73-75
18.	Gambling:	☐	☐	☐	76-78
				Ø M B P 2 9 0 2	01-08
19.	Alcoholism:	☐	☐	☐	19-21
20.	Religion:	☐	☐	☐	22-24
21.	Racial / cultural:	☐	☐	☐	25-27
22.	Drug abuse:	☐	☐	☐	28-30
23.	Self doubt / lack of confidence:	☐	☐	☐	31-33
24.	Abnormal fears:	☐	☐	☐	34-36
25.	Other: ____________	☐	☐	☐	37-39

Section 3 – Overall Evaluation

Taking into account all information you have obtained, what is the value of counselling in helping this patient?

0 = Same
1 = Worse
2 = Some improvement
3 = Marked improvement
4 = Complete resolution

☐ 40

Summary of Importance and Progress of Audit of Counselling

MIX
Papier aus verantwortungsvollen Quellen
Paper from responsible sources
FSC® C105338

If you have any concerns about our products,
you can contact us on
ProductSafety@springernature.com

In case Publisher is established outside the EU,
the EU authorized representative is:
Springer Nature Customer Service Center GmbH
Europaplatz 3, 69115 Heidelberg, Germany

Printed by Libri Plureos GmbH
in Hamburg, Germany